Praise for *The Heal Your Gut Cookbook*

"The GAPS Diet can change your life; the challenge is how to apply it. Hilary Boynton to the rescue! She is a busy mother of five and lives by the guiding principle of 'let your food be your medicine.' Along with photographer Mary Brackett, she has created this beautifully illustrated manual for creating delicious and nutritious GAPS meals. This book provides easy, mouthwatering recipes. It offers practical ways to restore your gut to optimum function and help you and your family take control of your gut health."

—**Dr. Joseph Mercola**, founder of Mercola.com

"If you think 'healing diet' means renunciation of delicious foods, you are in for a surprise. *The Heal Your Gut Cookbook* shows that you can enjoy every morsel while your body recovers from a lifetime of nutrient deficiencies and processed food. The recipes are delicious and the book beautifully illustrated. It is a wonderful contribution to the literature on the topic."

—**Sally Fallon Morell**, president of the Weston A. Price Foundation

"More than half of American children are currently diagnosed with a chronic illness, and much of that statistic can be attributed to a long list of damaging exposures (from antibiotics to GMOs) that have destroyed the health of the American gut. For all the damage we have done to our gut and immune health, there is hope. Healing the gut through nutrient-dense, restorative diets like the GAPS Diet is absolutely foundational to recovery. Recovery is within reach, and *The Heal Your Gut Cookbook* is a terrific companion for that journey."

—**Beth Lambert**, author of *A Compromised Generation: The Epidemic of Chronic Illness in America's Children*, executive director of Epidemic Answers and executive producer of The Canary Kids Project

"Over my many years of healing through diet, especially healing the gut through diet, the problem has always been how to make the information and the food readily available to those in need. In the beginning, the food was not to be had, and the diet plans, recipes, and explanations were not to be found. Over the years this has begun to change. There are ever-expanding farmers markets, small businesses, and cooperative ventures that are filling the food-availability gap. Hilary's and Mary's book is a valuable addition to the question of what to do with the food and why. This book is another small step in my eventual fading away, as I can finally say 'It's all out there now. Just follow the advice and wonderful recipes; my work is done.'"

—**Dr. Thomas Cowan**, author of *The Fourfold Path to Healing* and coauthor of *The Nourishing Traditions Book of Baby & Child Care*

"If you feel enslaved to standard food and pharmaceutical remedies, *The Heal Your Gut Cookbook* provides a comprehensive can-do liberation plan. These pages scream 'freedom to be healthy!' As a farmer servicing wellness-lovers, I yearn for the kind of understanding and participation a recipe roadmap like this can offer. Wellness eaters create wellness landscapes."

—**Joel Salatin**, Polyface Farm

"Hilary Boynton is a wife, mother of five, artist, amazing cook, health coach, and cooking teacher. She, along with Mary Brackett, has created a delectable cookbook, full of recipes that are very flavorful and yummy. *The Heal Your Gut Cookbook* is sure to be coveted by people on the GAPS Diet, as well as people looking for nutrient-dense, healthy, and delicious meals."

—**Kristin Canty**, director of *Farmageddon: The Unseen War on American Family Farms*

"I couldn't stop reading Hilary Boynton's and Mary Brackett's book on the GAPS diet, *The Heal Your Gut Cookbook*. I found myself famished for the amazing information and guidance they offer on how to improve gut health and ultimately restore optimum immune function. Hilary and Mary do a wonderful job of weaving their own personal and family stories of health redemption together with fantastic, mouth-watering recipes that build on Hilary's food philosophy. Moreover, the recipes are easy to follow. I plan to make this book available to my friends and family, so they can all benefit from the important information here."

—**David Gumpert**, author of *Life, Liberty, and the Pursuit of Food Rights* and *The Raw Milk Revolution*

"The GAPS protocol is a particularly effective antidote to the standard American diet. But GAPS involves a big lifestyle change and a serious commitment to cooking from scratch. This change can be intimidating, even to experienced home cooks. Hilary Boynton's and Mary Brackett's new book makes GAPS accessible to a wide audience, both through its no-nonsense narrative and through its wealth of straightforward, delicious, and healthy recipes. It's as if she is saying, 'You are not alone. . . and here's what we're having for dinner.' Anyone following GAPS, or even just thinking about it, will appreciate the recipes and ideas in this book."

—**Alex Lewin**, author of *Real Food Fermentation*

"Hilary is an excellent cook and has mastered the GAPS Diet for her family. If you want to try the GAPS Diet, this book is a must-have. Her recipes are simple, nourishing, and delicious."

—**Diana Rodgers**, author of *Paleo Lunches and Breakfasts on the Go*

"Hilary Boynton, busy and dedicated mother of five, has teamed with photographer extraordinaire Mary Brackett to create a beautiful book that accurately and elegantly lays out delicious, delightful, and fun recipes for the GAPS Diet. No one will be bored again while cooking to heal. The highest kudos to Hilary and Mary: *The Heal Your Gut Cookbook* is a true gift to all of us!"

—**Monica Corrado**, MA, CNC, traditional food chef, GAPS cooking teacher, and certified nutrition consultant

"As a homeopath, this is now my recommended go-to guide for my clients and students. Instead of explaining what they ought not to eat, I now direct them to this little masterpiece. It offers freedom from worry and is loaded with satisfying meals. A must-own!"

—**Joette Calabrese**, homeopathic consultant and author of *How to Raise a Drug-Free Family System*

the HEAL YOUR GUT cookbook

Nutrient-Dense Recipes for Intestinal Health Using the GAPS Diet

Hilary Boynton and Mary G. Brackett

Foreword by Dr. Natasha Campbell-McBride

Chelsea Green Publishing
White River Junction, Vermont

Developmental Editor: Brianne Goodspeed
Project Manager: Hillary Gregory
Copy Editor: Laura Jorstad
Proofreader: Eileen M. Clawson
Indexer: Peggy Holloway
Designer: Melissa Jacobson

Printed in the United States of America.
First printing August, 2014.
10 9 8 7 6 5 4   16 17 18 19 20

green press INITIATIVE

Chelsea Green Publishing is committed to preserving ancient forests and natural resources. We elected to print this title on paper containing at least 10% post-consumer recycled paper, processed chlorine-free. As a result, for this printing, we have saved:

38 Trees (40' tall and 6-8" diameter)
17,811 Gallons of Wastewater
17 million BTUs Total Energy
1,192 Pounds of Solid Waste
3,284 Pounds of Greenhouse Gases

Chelsea Green Publishing made this paper choice because we are a member of the Green Press Initiative, a nonprofit program dedicated to supporting authors, publishers, and suppliers in their efforts to reduce their use of fiber obtained from endangered forests. For more information, visit www.greenpressinitiative.org.

Environmental impact estimates were made using the Environmental Defense Paper Calculator. For more information visit: www.papercalculator.org.

Our Commitment to Green Publishing

Chelsea Green sees publishing as a tool for cultural change and ecological stewardship. We strive to align our book manufacturing practices with our editorial mission and to reduce the impact of our business enterprise in the environment. We print our books and catalogs on chlorine-free recycled paper, using vegetable-based inks whenever possible. This book may cost slightly more because it was printed on paper that contains recycled fiber, and we hope you'll agree that it's worth it. Chelsea Green is a member of the Green Press Initiative (www.greenpressinitiative .org), a nonprofit coalition of publishers, manufacturers, and authors working to protect the world's endangered forests and conserve natural resources. *The Heal Your Gut Cookbook* was printed on paper supplied by QuadGraphics that contains at least 10% postconsumer recycled fiber.

Library of Congress Cataloging-in-Publication Data
Boynton, Hilary.
  The heal your gut cookbook : nutrient-dense recipes for intestinal health using the GAPS diet / Hilary Boynton and Mary G. Brackett ; foreword by Natasha Campbell-McBride.
      pages cm
  Includes bibliographical references and index.
  ISBN 978-1-60358-561-3 (paperback) — ISBN 978-1-60358-562-0 (ebook)
1. Gastrointestinal system—Diseases—Diet therapy. 2. Cooking for the sick. I. Brackett, Mary G. II. Title.
  RC816.B736 2014
  641.5'631—dc23
                    2014018958

Chelsea Green Publishing
85 North Main Street, Suite 120
White River Junction, VT 05001
(802) 295-6300
www.chelseagreen.com

MIX
Paper from
responsible sources
FSC® C084269

With love and gratitude to my five beautiful children: Dossie, Cooper, Campbell, Wyatt, and Tanner. And to my amazing husband, Nick: You make it so much fun! —HB

To my Loves: Chris, the greatest partner a girl could ask for, thank you for being my inspiration, my cheerleader, my second opinion, and my rock throughout this wild (and delicious!) journey; and to Chet, the most amazing gift to have been bestowed upon my life . . . your life gives my life purpose. I love you both more than you will ever know. —MGB

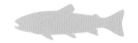

Contents

Foreword

Mothers are my heroes! A mother's love can overcome anything! This recipe book was created by two such heroes. Taking your family through the GAPS Nutritional Protocol and working through individual health problems takes a huge determination, self-discipline, and love. Then to share with the world what you have learned on the way, in order to help others to make this journey with more ease, is an act of kindness and generosity. The world can only be grateful to Hilary Boynton and Mary Brackett for this work! The recipes are wonderful, with beautiful pictures, and the book is full of useful tips and helpful guidance and inspiration. I thoroughly recommend it.

The concept of GAPS (Gut and Psychology Syndrome and Gut and Physiology Syndrome) establishes a connection between the state of the person's digestive system and the health of the rest of the body. We live in a world of growing epidemics of mental and physical illness. These epidemics are underlined by another big epidemic, which is increasingly recognized as the cause of those illnesses. This big epidemic is abnormal gut flora or gut dysbiosis. Recent research has established that around 90 percent of all cells and genetic material in the human body is our gut flora—myriad microbes that live inside our digestive systems. In order to be healthy, a person has to have a healthy gut flora dominated by beneficial species of microbes. In our modern world where people are regularly taking antibiotics and other pharmaceutical drugs, where food is laced with chemicals alien to the human physiology, an increasing number of people have damaged, abnormal gut flora dominated by pathogenic microbes. As a result, a person's gut is unable to nourish the body properly; instead it produces large amounts of toxins that absorb into the bloodstream, get spread around the body, and cause disease. This is GAPS. To understand this concept fully please read my book on this subject.

The list of GAPS conditions is long; I divided them into two groups:

1. Gut and Psychology Syndrome
2. Gut and Physiology Syndrome

Gut and Psychology Syndrome, or GAPS, includes learning disabilities and mental disorders such as ADHD/ADD, dyslexia, dyspraxia, autism, addictions, depression, obsessive-compulsive disorder, bipolar disorder, schizophrenia, epilepsy, eating disorders, and many other conditions, which stem from abnormal function of the brain. Many of these conditions have no established diagnostic labels and present themselves as a mixture of various so-called mental symptoms: mood alterations, memory and cognitive problems, behavioral and social problems, panic attacks, anxiety, involuntary movements, various tics and fits, sensory problems, sleep problems, and so on.

Gut and Physiology Syndrome, also known as GAPS, includes various chronic physical conditions that stem from an unhealthy gut, such as autoimmune conditions (celiac disease, rheumatoid arthritis, diabetes type one, multiple sclerosis, amyotrophic lateral sclerosis, systemic lupus erythematosus, osteoarthritis, Crohn's disease, ulcerative colitis, autoimmune skin problems, chronic cystitis, nephropathy, neuropathy, et cetera), asthma, eczema, allergies, chronic fatigue syndrome, fibromyalgia, myalgic encephalomyelitis, multiple chemical sensitivity, arthritis, PMS and other menstrual problems, endocrine disorders (thyroid, adrenal, and other), and digestive disorders (irritable bowel syndrome, gastritis, colitis, and so forth). Many conditions do not fit into any diagnostic box and can present as a mixture of symptoms: digestive problems, fatigue, muscular weakness, cramps and abnormal muscle tone, pain and ache in joints and muscles, skin problems, neurological and hormonal abnormalities.

In almost every person the symptoms from both GAP Syndromes overlap: People with mental problems suffer physical symptoms (painful joints and muscles, fatigue, skin problems, asthma, hormonal problems, autoimmunity), while people with physical problems have mental symptoms (such as depression, "brain fog," inability to concentrate, mood swings, sleep abnormalities, memory problems, anxiety, tremors, tics, fits, and more). When the digestive system is unwell, instead of being a source of nourishment it becomes a major source of toxicity in the body; nothing in the body can function well. Any organ, any system, any cell can show symptoms of distress—usually most of them respond with some symptoms. As a result GAPS patients are often the most difficult (if not impossible) for mainstream medicine to fathom and to help. The GAPS Nutritional Protocol is designed to treat all of those conditions starting from the roots.

Our digestive system holds the roots of our health. If those roots are not healthy, then the rest of the body cannot be healthy. So the treatment of any chronic disease has to start from the gut. The human gut is a long tube; what you fill that tube with has a direct effect on its well-being. Food—the person's daily diet—is the number one treatment for any chronic disease, and the GAPS Diet is the most important part of the GAPS Nutritional Protocol. This book will help you to implement the GAPS Diet by providing you with a large variety of delicious recipes and ideas of how to serve food. It is the recipes that make any diet an enjoyable experience. I have no doubt that even a complete novice to cooking will become an expert cook after having followed advice in this book!

—Dr. Natasha Campbell-McBride, MD, author of
Gut and Psychology Syndrome, Revised and Expanded Edition

Introduction

Hilary's Story

Looking back, it all makes perfect sense. Wow, if I had only known then what I know now. But if that were the case, I wouldn't be writing this book. I guess things really do happen for a reason.

Starting in high school, I lived completely "fat-free" for nearly a decade. During that time, years of playing intense Division One soccer (and having way too much fun in college) ultimately taxed my body to the brink. The cumulative effect of burning so much energy and then "replenishing" with bagels, pasta, cereal, and Butter Buds really did a doozy on my gut health. Not to mention being on the birth control pill and Accutane for bad skin.

I had no idea of the damage done until I was plagued by infertility as a young newlywed, which was quite possibly the most painful thing I'd ever endured. Why, at twenty-six, was I not able to carry a baby? Well, I think I know the answer to that now: I was malnourished. After years of trying, though, I was finally abundantly blessed, with triplets! Two boys and a girl. However, these blessings came with the help of modern intervention, not due to improved heath, I'm sorry to say.

Along with the stress of new motherhood, my poor eating habits continued when—boom!—I got pregnant again. How could it be? Surely it wouldn't stick; I had been on birth control pills again for the past three years. Well, the excitement of having conceived naturally must have worked some kind of magic, because that baby was here to stay. But shortly after his arrival, the scratching began: He was an eczema baby. Itchy, fussy, and breaking my heart. Months of sleepless nights kept me searching for answers. What had caused this? And how could it be treated? As my desperate quest for answers continued, I found myself pregnant again. What the . . . ? Had I even had sex in the past six months with four babies under three? Well, that little guy hung in there, too, and now we had five blessings under our roof. But still, my son's eczema flared.

One day, a year later, the answer finally came. I was at the grocery store with kids in tow, trying to make good choices for my family. If the label said ORGANIC, I assumed it was okay. Crackers, yogurt, fruit snacks. When I ran into an old friend, the film director and farm advocate Kristin Canty, I told her about my now-toddler's continuing plight. She gave me a recommendation that would change my life forever.

"You should try giving him raw milk."

Huh? What was raw milk? Did she mean . . . unpasteurized? Certainly that could not be good for us. But I was at my wit's end, so I went for it. And guess what? It worked! The eczema was subdued, with real food alone! So this is where my journey began.

Overcome with gratitude and amazement, I wanted to learn more and share the information. I attended conferences: Weston A. Price, Paleo, and the Fourfold Path to Healing. I purged our pantry and fridge: out with the cereals and skim milk, in with the raw milk and pastured eggs. Life was changing, and for five years we were great. No major sicknesses, and no trips to the doctor.

However, it takes time to undo the years of poor choices I had made in the past. Various problems began cropping up: My daughter Dossie with petit mal epilepsy, three kids with speech delays, and now, enamel was not forming correctly on my eczema baby's teeth (with seven cavities to boot). But outwardly my kids seemed healthy, so how could this be? They were never sick, and I fed them all nutrient-dense foods. Could it be related to their gut health?

When I heard Natasha Campbell-McBride speak at a Weston A. Price conference in the fall of 2012, I began to sense that it was time to take the nutrient-dense diet one step further. I read everything I could about GAPS. I scoured the web for information, inspiration, and confirmation. But I was overwhelmed and anxious. There were "stages" and restrictions. What exactly can we eat, and when? What can't we eat, and why? How would I prepare meals that my kids and husband would actually eat? I dreaded starting the diet because I knew that it was strict, and that there would be a lot of moving pieces with such a large family. I wondered if I had the brain power to not only learn everything there was to learn about GAPS, but put the diet into practice as well. And I expected doubts, if not downright refusal, from my husband, kids, and extended family.

But I was desperately searching for a way to manage Dossie's seizures. In March 2013, one of my clients introduced me to a medical intuitive named Laura Graye. My husband was skeptical and concerned at the amount of money I was spending as I investigated holistic therapies, so I asked Laura if she would consider meeting us to explain what she did before we invested money in yet another alternative treatment. She drove to our home, spent two hours with us at no charge, and—after looking at us and hearing our stories—said she was convinced that the GAPS Diet was our answer. She pulled out her markers and a dry erase board and proceeded to diagram a healthy gut and an unhealthy gut (see the sidebar "All Diseases Begin in the Gut" on page 3). My previously skeptical husband and I started the GAPS Diet the next day.

When we jumped into GAPS feetfirst, I started collecting, adapting, and creating recipes. I took notes about what the kids loved (and what they hated). I kept track of how everyone was doing, feeling, pooping, and sleeping and developed strategies for eating out, having sleepovers, and going to birthday parties.

I'm happy to say that we all adapted with minimal fuss, and here's the best part: After nearly a year on the diet, we weaned Dossie completely off Depakote. She is presently weaning off Zarontin as well, her second of three seizure medications. As for our eczema baby, he is free and clear of symptoms, and there have never been any signs of the predicted allergies or asthma. Not to mention that we've survived two consecutive brutal New England winters without one trip to the doctor! Believe me, I don't take for granted the blessing of having not one but five strong, healthy children who are adventurous eaters. I count each blessing every day.

The other immense gift of the GAPS Diet is that it has empowered me to "go with my gut." I have always sought the approval of others, seeking reassurance and endorsement for everything I do. How often as a new mother did I run to the doctor's office for absolutely every little thing? The GAPS Diet gave me the power to have a direct impact on my own healing and that of my loved ones. It has made me a stronger person because I've often had to stand up to naysayers and their notions of "normal." Most important, it has taught our family to tune in to the subtle wisdom of our bodies as the ultimate authority.

Mary's Story

It's hard to say exactly when my story began, because like so many Americans of my generation, my poor health started well before I was born. I was the fifth and last child born into the Giordano clan just outside Boston in the early '80s. My sibling Mark, born just three years prior to my arrival, was premature and didn't survive more than a few minutes past birth. My mother, like most middle-class women of the time, was simply following along with the dietary trends of the age, feeding herself and her family from the burgeoning selection of processed foods, rancid fats, and pesticide-laden fresh vegetables and fruits. Little did she know that her own health was in danger from the nutrient depletion of a poor diet and carrying so many children. When her own doctor told her to abort what turned out to be me, she found herself a new doctor. I was born via emergency C-section in early September 1982. Thus began my fight for life, for answers, and for health.

As a child I was always sick. Back then our local pediatrician practiced out of his home just up the road from us. He became such a figure in my young life, because I was always in his office! Ear infections, strep throat, flu, colds, viruses, chicken pox, ovarian cysts, mono—you name it, I had it. My health woes peaked when I was diagnosed at sixteen with an "unidentifiable virus." I lost fourteen pounds in two weeks, because everything I ate made my stomach burn in writhing pain. From there, life was a revolving door at the hospital. Two and a half years and thousands of dollars later, my doctors gave me a diagnosis of irritable bowel syndrome and sent me on my way. At that time there was no protocol for healing; the attitude was "good luck, don't let the door hit you on the way out."

Sickness always waited at my doorstep, along with anxiety and depression. As a young person in today's world, I simply couldn't cut it. In 2008, completely desperate and exhausted from every failed attempt to be healthy, I switched doctors for the fourth time in five years. I pleaded with my new doctor to figure out the root of all my health woes, not just how to manage my symptoms. He ran a series of blood tests, which showed that I was "fine" and then showed me the door. Enraged at the lack of care and understanding, I switched doctors (again!) and vowed to get to the bottom of what was wrong with me, uncover what systems in my body were broken, and actually heal them.

The universe has a funny way of opening itself up to you when you need it, and as serendipity would have it I learned of the Weston A. Price Foundation just days after leaving my doctor's office. It certainly made sense that real foods— vegetables, meats, and (gasp!) fats—should be the basis of our diet. I'd been a vegetarian off and on for many years and was reluctant to give up my beliefs, but I knew something had to give. And so it began: my slow road off the Standard American Diet.

The years that followed were full of trial and error. I learned that although a food might be nourishing to one person, it could damage another. After years of being told to "listen to your doctor" for answers, it took me a while to learn to listen to my own body to determine what was actually my medicine and my poison. Not only that, but I had to reprioritize my life in order to afford real food. I learned that Americans spent approximately 43 percent of their income on food in 1900, versus an average of only 13 percent spent today. Processed food is incredibly cheap; food that is produced using time-honored traditions in farming and animal husbandry is not. And although I still have moments when it pains me to part with a solid chunk of cash for vegetables and meats, I remind myself of the nutritional investment I am making.

A few years into my health food journey, my son Chet was born. Within a month of his arrival, his doctors found blood in his stool. They informed me I had to come off all allergens— milk, eggs, soy, nuts, shellfish, and gluten (which I had already eliminated for myself). As a new mother in the throes of sleep deprivation and starvation, I became completely spooked by food. I foolishly decided that becoming a raw vegan was the way to go. After a short period of health, I began to feel my body breaking down once again. I entered a painful and dark time when I constantly felt awful, physically, emotionally, spiritually; I was broken and hopeless.

In late winter of 2011, I met Hilary in Wayland, Massachusetts, at a Holistic Moms meeting, a casual monthly meeting for holistic-minded mamas. Hilary presented information on nutrient-dense foods and the Weston A. Price

Foundation. She extended an invitation to one of her cooking classes, which I gratefully accepted. There I realized that this was how I needed to eat, but I had a hard time with a lot of ingredients, namely milk, butter, and eggs. I shared my story with a fellow student and was stunned to learn her experiences were similar to mine. She mentioned the GAPS Diet and her successes with it, so naturally I went home to research it. Within a week I had switched my family's diet to Full GAPS, where we stayed for six months as I learned to cook and worked up the courage to begin the GAPS Introduction Diet. (Because my gut was so compromised at that point, I was concerned that the introductory portion of the diet would leave me bedridden as the toxins left my body—which happens to many people who go from the Standard American Diet right into the Intro Diet. I also needed to prepare myself for the limited food choices and the idea of eating for health, and health alone.) After a short time on the Intro Diet, I noticed that some foods still gave me stomach pain, so I recorded everything I ate—a key component in learning to see what works in your own body and what doesn't.

Unfortunately, after starting the Intro Diet, I experienced major stomach distension from eating a bowl of butternut squash soup and ended up looking four months' pregnant! It didn't make any sense. I started going to a functional medicine doctor (a doctor who seeks out the root causes of illness) for both myself and my son. A slew of tests revealed that I had fructose malabsorption, virtually no hydrochloric acid in my stomach, and serious yeast overgrowth. The GAPS Diet helped me uncover these underlying issues in my gastrointestinal tract. The protocol for healing in my life and that of my son is different from that of Hilary and her family. So although I completely advocate for the GAPS Diet, I learned that my body won't thrive on it if there are underlying issues such as yeast overgrowth, parasites, small intestinal bacterial overgrowth (SIBO), fructose malabsorption, or lack of hydrochloric acid (HCL), digestive enzymes, or bile acids. Once those issues are recognized and addressed, the GAPS Diet can heal and seal your gut as it was intended to do.

My story is intended not to discourage you, but to give you an idea of what is happening if you are following GAPS and still not healing. It is discouraging and upsetting to spend vast amounts of time, energy, and money on a diet that isn't working. Take heed: It will work, but you may need to do a few things first. My advice is to make judicious records of what you are eating and the subsequent symptoms you experience, then seek out a functional medicine team (medical doctor, registered dietitian, and/or naturopathic doctor). If you are anything like me and have experienced gut dysbiosis for years, you may need to undergo various tests to determine what underlying issues you need to address before even starting on GAPS.

Here in 2014, I am happy to say that this is the best I've ever felt in my life. The stomach pain, anxiety, and depression that once plagued me have all but disappeared. My little man, Chet, is a happy and healthy three-year-old who thrives on real, whole foods. The GAPS Diet helped me uncover an abundance of joy and gratitude for life that I never knew possible.

This book is a labor of love; both Hilary and I hope that it serves you as a reference for truly remarkable health. As you embark on this journey, know that it may be frustrating and lonely at times, as going against the grain often is, but know also that you *will* heal. You can regain your health through patience, determination, and love in your heart. As insurance premiums skyrocket and many of our loved ones fall ill due to the frankenfoods we have allowed into our lives, awareness of how our gut health controls the health of our bodies will grow. Have faith that you're doing the right thing and know that you're not alone.

Authors' Note

Although *The Heal Your Gut Cookbook* is a labor of love for both of us, Mary and I decided, for simplicity's sake, that the book would tell my story, while visual inspiration comes courtesy of Mary's beautiful photographs.

—Hilary Boynton

Before You Begin the GAPS Diet

The GAPS Diet is based on the principle that what we consume affects the health of our gut, and in turn what nutrients are absorbed into our bodies and what toxins stay out. In this way, gut function affects just about every function of the body. The GAPS Diet is specifically designed to heal digestive issues and disorders, and to ameliorate any conditions that might be related. It is a restricted (but delicious) program that will promote the healing and sealing of a compromised gut lining—commonly referred to as leaky gut—so that individuals with related illnesses, psychological and physical, can improve their health. It was conceived by Dr. Natasha Campbell-McBride as an evolution of the Specific Carbohydrate Diet by Dr. Sydney Valentine Haas, which was then popularized by Elaine Gottschall in her book *Breaking the Vicious Cycle*.

The GAPS Diet occurs in two phases. The Introduction Diet lasts eighteen to thirty days (roughly three to five days per stage) and involves removing all foods that might be gut irritants, such as dairy, from your daily intake. You then reintroduce certain foods slowly and look for adverse reactions. (This can include stomach pain, hand flapping, seizures, eczema, and the like.) If you're already comfortable in the kitchen and currently eat a whole-foods diet, starting with the Introduction Diet may not be such an adjustment for you. However, if you tend to eat more processed foods, consider giving yourself a little time on Full GAPS first so that you can wean yourself off the sugar, salt, fillers, and stabilizers your body has come to crave. Once you begin to feel familiar and comfortable with the foods allowed

Begin at the Beginning: The GAPS Sourcebook

Before you embark on the GAPS Diet, it is essential that you read Dr. Natasha Campbell-McBride's *Gut and Psychology Syndrome*, Revised and Expanded Edition, to understand this nutritional protocol and its application as a natural treatment for autism, ADD/ADHD, Crohn's disease, celiac disease, dyslexia, dyspraxia, depression, schizophrenia, and other chronic illnesses. The GAPS Diet is complex, and we cannot overstress the importance of reading Dr. Campbell-McBride's work.

during each stage of the GAPS Introduction Diet, you may feel more ready to launch into the Intro. The Full GAPS Diet is the main portion of the diet and should last at least two years for maximum restoration of gut health. It includes a wide selection of foods that can be prepared simply and are easy to digest. Enjoying Full GAPS after the restrictions of the Intro Diet is like feasting every day.

Most of us are not mindful of the importance of gut health, or just how far we in the modern world have been distanced from it. Many of us were not breast-fed; we received countless simultaneous vaccinations as children and were overprescribed antibiotics and medications from the start. Any one of these phenomena could contribute to an early imbalance of gut flora—not to mention subsequent years of consuming processed foods, artificial sweeteners, genetically modified foods, and heavily sprayed produce! Well, the notion of gut health is finally entering the mainstream. This is ironic, since Hippocrates, the father of modern medicine (460–370 BC), warned long ago, "All diseases begin in the gut."

At birth, a mother's gut flora is passed on to her baby. Good or bad, the baby gets what it gets. Think of your great-grandmother's flora compared to yours. She was most likely breast-fed, with no obsessive hand sanitizing, GMOs, antibiotics, or drugs. Now, simply by being members of modern society, we have unknowingly diminished the birthright of our gut flora; over the past few generations, its quality and balance are believed to have deteriorated significantly. Today there are diseases that did not exist fifty years ago. Think of the diseases that will plague the next generation, and generations to come. We are facing an epidemic.

Still, if we adopt a glass-half-full attitude, we have an opportunity to turn things around. What's done is done and we can't go back, but think of the gift we can give to our children and grandchildren. We must all learn how to cook again! We must pass along nutritional lessons learned through recipes and the loving act of preparing a meal. It's as simple as that. Although this book describes a diet designed to support special needs, it's also a valuable resource for everyone, crafted in celebration of our ancestors' traditional diets. Here you'll learn the basics of stocking your pantry, planning a meal, and working in the kitchen; most important, you'll come to enjoy and celebrate your own home cooking.

There is time and effort involved; the GAPS Diet is rigorous, but like anything, it gets easier with time and practice. The goal is worth it: your family's perfect health. Dr. Weston A. Price discovered that this is possible in the 1930s when he was researching indigenous, nonindustrialized cultures who were eating whole foods—and living free from much disease. We cannot control everything in our environment, of course, but we do have a say in what we feed ourselves.

All Diseases Begin in the Gut

Laura Graye, MS, CEM

Approximately 88 percent of our body's immunity is found in the lining of our gastrointestinal (GI) system. Its positioning there is primarily to stop invaders from moving out of the digestive tract into the body. Over time, without the beneficial bacteria and proper balance in the gut, toxins, opportunistic bacteria, and parasites chisel away at the physical barrier wall and can create leaky gut. Once there is an opening in the wall lining, pathogens escape from the GI, travel through the bloodstream, penetrate the blood–brain barrier, and wreak havoc on the specific functions of our cells, causing any number of diseases. What causes a healthy gut to become imbalanced? Poor diet, antibiotic use, low digestive enzymes, alkalinity, acidity, chemical toxins, environmental toxins, radiation, blood sugar irregularity, stress, and pregnancy- and birth-inherited gut imbalances.

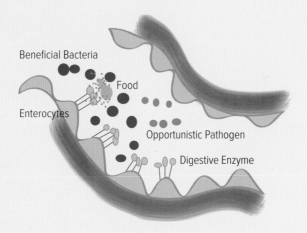

A healthy gut has an approximate ratio of 8:2 of beneficial bacteria to opportunistic bacteria. The beneficial bacteria feed on certain types of opportunistic fungi (candida and the like), create an internal wall of defense against pathogens escaping the intestine, and help digest foods to be transformed into energy.

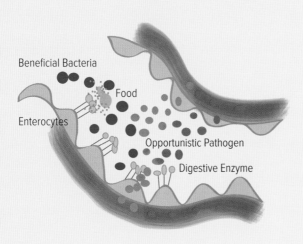

When the proper ratio is out of balance, the beneficial bacteria can no longer protect the walls of the gut. Pathogens, including opportunistic bacteria, wear down the enterocytes and break through the intestinal lining. Having escaped the gastrointestinal system, the pathogens now enter the bloodstream as antigens. There they create an autoimmune response, attack cells, break through the blood–brain barrier, and create an environment conducive to disease.

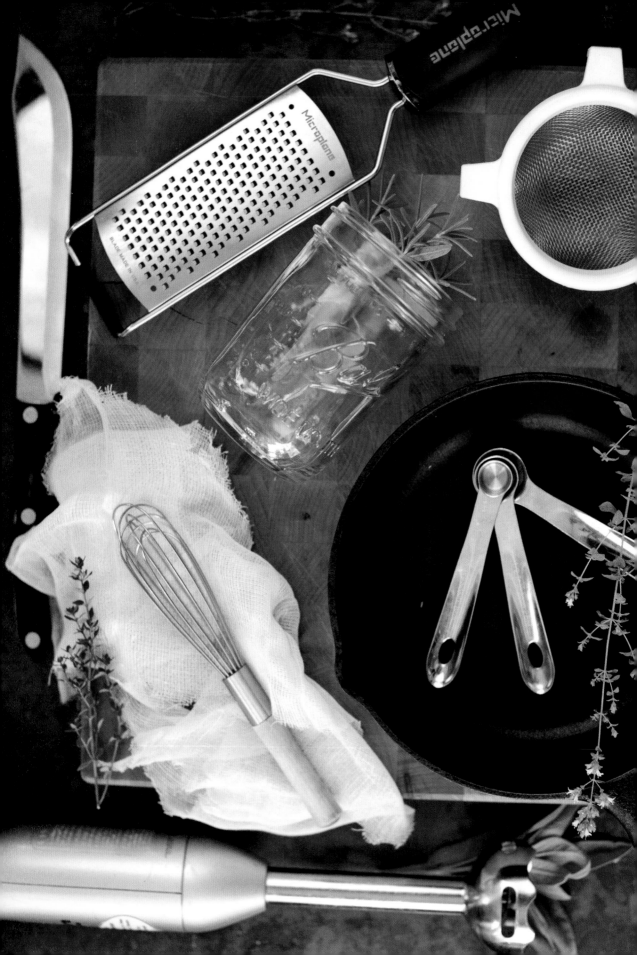

Though not required, the following utensils and tools are helpful when you are following the GAPS Diet.

Slow cooker/Crock-Pot
VitaClay (see resources)
Blender/Vitamix
Juicer
Immersion blender
Sharp knives
Food processor
Measuring cups and spoons
Cookie sheets/jelly-roll pans
Stainless-steel pots and pans
Nut milk bags
Dehydrator
Teflex dehydrator sheets
Metal or glass straws
Gallon ziplock bags
Parchment paper
Tupperware
Thermoses (Klean Kanteen)
Reusable water bottles
  (Klean Kanteen)

To-go reusable containers
Salt and pepper grinders
Widemouthed jars/Bormioli Rocco
  or Ball jars
Grolsch bottles for fermented
  drinks
Garlic press
Ladle
Strainers, large-mesh and
  fine-mesh
Cheesecloth
Labels
Water filter system or attachments
Cast-iron pan
Zester
Grater
Canning funnel
Pyrex liquid measuring cup
Fun soup bowls

Filtered Water

Due to toxins such as chlorine and fluoride in the water supply, we recommend that you always use filtered water while on the GAPS Diet. Although chlorine, for example, is effective at killing any pathogenic microbes that may be in your water supply, it also kills the good bacteria in your gut! A reverse-osmosis filter is a great option. A quick Google search should give you plenty of price points to consider.

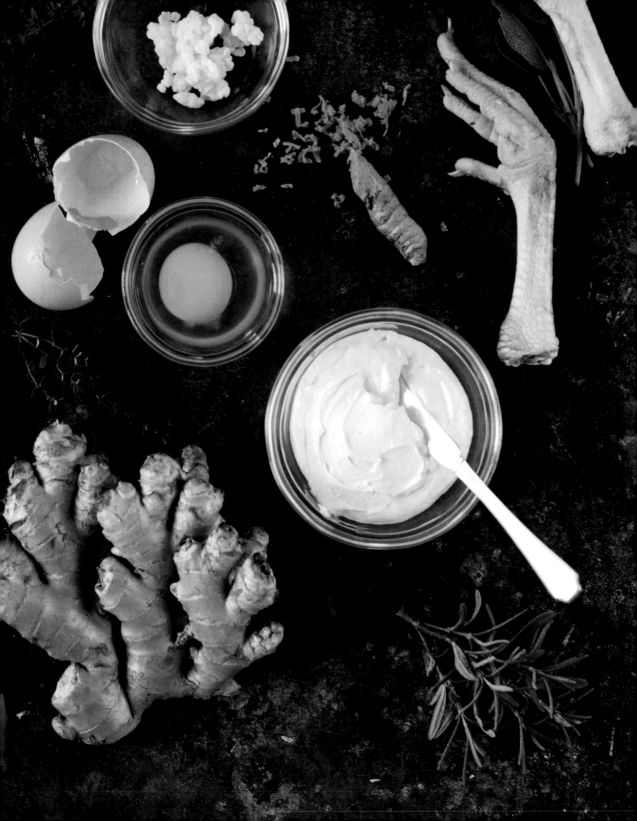

Stocking the Larder

When you start stocking your larder, be sure to get the best ingredients you can find. Organic, pastured, and farm-fresh is always best. It may take a little investigating to find all your sources for good reliable food, but once you do it will be easy to stock up on supplies that will last for months. An extra fridge and/or freezer can be helpful, especially if you are trying to be economical and buy in bulk. A local Weston A. Price Foundation chapter leader can help you source the best ingredients in your area.

Unrefined sea salt
Organic spices
Raw nuts, seeds, and nut and
   seed butters
Organic pastured eggs
Organic pastured chicken and pork
100 percent grass-fed beef and lamb
Chicken heads and feet
Sugar-free bacon
Organic coconut oil
Red palm oil
Ghee
Sesame oil
Cold-pressed olive oil
Pastured lard, beef tallow, lamb
   tallow, duck fat
Herbal teas
Coffee substitute (I like
   Dandy Blend)
Kefir grains
Bone broth and meat stock:
   chicken, beef, and fish
Great Lakes Gelatin
Raw honey
Fermented vegetables
Bragg's Apple Cider Vinegar

Coconut vinegar
Whey
Sauerkraut or pickle juice
Fresh fruits and vegetables
Whole raw milk to make yogurt
   and kefir
Whole raw cream to culture and
   make butter
Raw cultured butter
Coconut aminos (a soy-free
   seasoning sauce)
Shredded coconut flakes, large
   and small
Dried fruit
Unprocessed homemade
   condiments
Almond and
   homemade coconut flour
Roasted carob or
   raw unsweetened cacao powder
Full-fat coconut milk
Pure vanilla extract
Onions
Garlic
Squash
Fresh ginger and turmeric

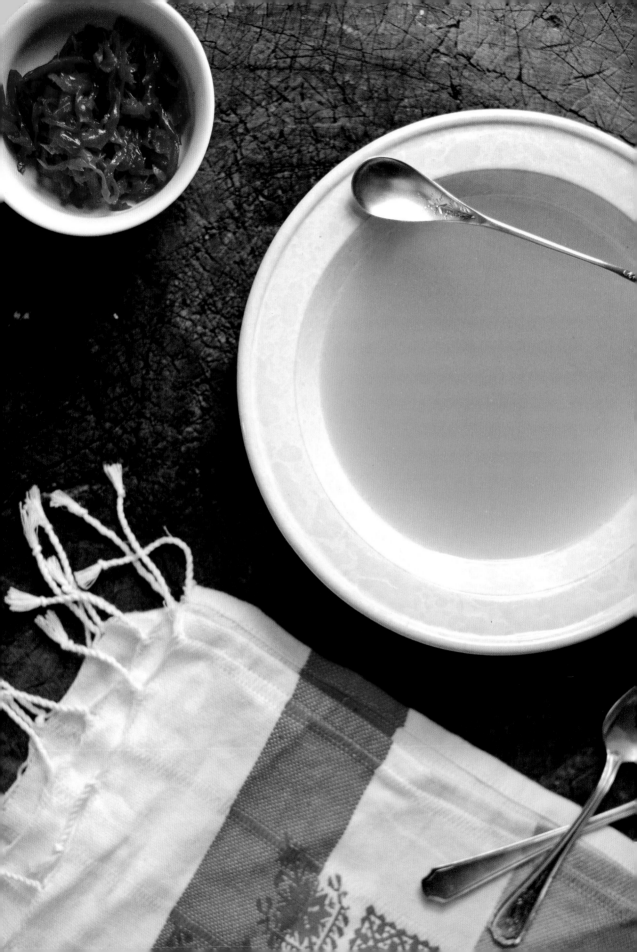

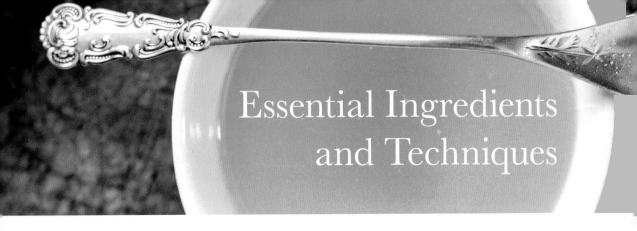

Essential Ingredients and Techniques

The following pages are intended to help you understand and master some essential cooking techniques that you'll be using on the GAPS Diet. Familiarize yourself with this section and its recipes. They will become the basis of many soups, condiments, snacks, and treats and will give you a foundation to develop your own variations. Once you become comfortable with these techniques, you'll gain confidence and find yourself creating original masterpieces on a regular basis! Some recipes in this section include ingredients that aren't allowed until later stages of the diet, so be sure to cross-reference the list of allowed foods on each stage before introducing these to your diet.

Meat Stock and Bone Broth

Boy, was I surprised to learn that there's a difference between meat stock and bone broth. Say what? In the fall of 2013, I was perusing the booths at a Weston A. Price Wise Traditions Conference when I came upon The Brothery's booth. The Flavor Chef, as he called himself, had set out samples of his (GAPS-friendly) 2-Hour Stock alongside a "regular bone broth." Wait a minute! What the heck? Here I was writing a GAPS cookbook and had no idea what the distinction was. Thank heavens for Monica Corrado, a GAPS cooking instructor and certified nutrition consultant, whose booth was nearby and who also happened to have our manuscript in hand, vetting all the recipes. I quickly asked her to tell me what a two-hour stock is and why we needed one. So hold on to your hats, folks, and read below straight from the horse's mouth. Monica to the rescue!

Meat Stock:
The Secret to Thriving Throughout the Intro Diet
Monica Corrado, MA, CNC

What is meat stock? What is bone broth? Aren't they the same? No, they are not. Meat stock is made by cooking pieces of meat that have a joint in them—such as turkey legs or thighs, a whole chicken cut up, or a beef or lamb shank—for a relatively short amount of time. Bone broth is cooked longer. Meat stock is cooked for an hour and a half to three hours for poultry and no more than six hours for beef, bison, or lamb unless you're using a slow cooker that will cook low and slow for a slightly longer period of time. Making it is making a meal: You will eat the meat, the cartilage or tendons, and the vegetables, and you'll drink the stock. It is the foundation of the Intro Diet, and knowing how to make it will help you get through it with ease.

Meat stock is milder in flavor than bone broth and has a different profile of amino acids (specifically glycine and proline), which is why it's used through the intro portion of the GAPS Diet. Individuals with gut issues often have brain function issues as well, which can be set off by the high concentration of glutamic acid and free glutamates in bone broth. Serving meat stock throughout the Intro Diet for those prone to seizures, tics, or ADD, or on the autism spectrum, can prevent these flares.

However, both meat stocks and bone broths are healing foods. Gelatin, found in the joints and knuckles of bones, is one of the most prominent "super foods" for healing a leaky gut. It protects and heals the mucosal lining of the digestive tract and helps to regenerate cells. It also aids in the digestion and absorption of nutrients. Marrow, found in the larger bones such as the femur, helps to strengthen bones and connective tissues and supports the immune system. Other healing properties promote the development and repair of healthy joints, ligaments, tendons, and bones, as well as hair and skin.

Basic Meat Stock: Turkey or Chicken Thighs or Quarters
Serves 4

2–3 pounds pastured turkey or chicken
   thighs or quarters, skin on
3–4 carrots, coarsely chopped
1 small onion, quartered
3–4 celery ribs, chopped

Handful of black peppercorns
1–2 teaspoons sea salt
2–3 sprigs fresh rosemary or thyme
2–4 tablespoons tomato paste (optional)
2–4 garlic cloves, to finish

Place all of the ingredients except the garlic in a 5- to 6-quart Dutch oven. Cover with water, to 2 inches above the ingredients. Place in a 350°F oven for 3 hours or in a Crock-Pot on low for 6 to 8 hours. Serve the meat and vegetables with a cup of stock alongside. Use a garlic press to add a small clove of garlic to each cup of stock, along with some good sea salt, whey, or probiotic juice.

Note: *You can also use a whole pastured chicken, cut up, in place of thighs or quarters.*

Basic Meat Stock: Beef, Bison, or Lamb
Serves 4

2–3 pounds grass-fed beef, bison, or lamb shanks
3–4 carrots, coarsely chopped
1 small onion, quartered
3–4 celery ribs, chopped

Handful of black peppercorns
1–2 teaspoons sea salt
2–3 sprigs fresh rosemary or thyme
2–4 tablespoons tomato paste (optional)
2–4 garlic cloves, to finish

Place all of the ingredients except the garlic in a 5- to 6-quart Dutch oven. Cover with water, to 2 inches above the ingredients. Place in the oven at 350°F for no longer than 6 to 8 hours or in a Crock-Pot on low for 8 to 10 hours. (Lamb requires less time than beef or bison.) Serve the meat and vegetables with a cup of stock alongside. Use a garlic press to add a small clove of garlic to each cup of stock, along with some good sea salt, whey, or probiotic juice.

Note: *Once you're on Full GAPS, you may wish to brown the meat in lard, tallow, ghee, or another healthy fat as a first step in making meat stock.*

The beauty of meat stock is not only that you make your stock and get a meal to eat to boot, but also that you can do wonders with the leftovers. This is truly an efficient way to make stock for this diet! Here are a few options for leftovers:

- Reheat what you have made and eat the same meal again.
- Pick the meat off the bones, save the bones in a freezer bag in the freezer to make bone broth later (see page 12), place the meat back into the pot—and you now have stew. You may need to add a few more cooked vegetables, depending on how many you ate the first time!
- After picking the meat off the bones as described above, make a soup by adding more stock to the pot. Again, you may wish to add more vegetables.
- Strain the stock and reserve it in the refrigerator to drink later or to use as the basis of a vegetable soup. Pull the meat off the bones, saving the bones as above. You can make a meat salad with homemade mayonnaise (see page 107); make gravy with stock and gelatin and serve with cauliflower rice (see page 87); or use the meat for another entrée (see the "Poultry" and "Meat" chapters).

The Time-Honored Tradition
of Homemade Bone Broth

Bone broth is made from bones with a little bit of meat on them, which you cook for longer than you would a meat stock. You can introduce bone broths into your diet once you're through the Intro Diet and following Full GAPS. It's a good idea to prepare a large quantity of broth at a time; use it to make healthy soups, stews, and casseroles or simply to drink throughout the day as a beverage, complete with probiotic juice, good fat, and mineral-rich salt. What a wonder drug! Occasionally, when I say to a person who is sick, "You need some homemade bone broth," they look at me as if I'm crazy—like it's some foreign, exotic food. Yet this humble staple is perhaps the most traditional, nourishing, and nutrient-dense food available. It's also dirt-cheap to make. It does take a little time and effort, but once you get the hang of it, you will be movin' and groovin'.

Be sure to source your bones carefully. The best bones are from 100 percent grass-fed and -finished cows, pastured chickens, and wild-caught fish. Of course, you can make bone broth with lamb, turkey, bison, and venison bones, too. Just be sure that the livestock was raised to your standards. The best way to ensure excellent quality is to seek out a local, sustainable farmer, or to find a reputable resource online.

It took me a few years to work up the courage to order chicken feet from our co-op, and another year after that to order chicken heads. These are not ingredients we are used to seeing in the average American grocery store! Nonetheless, they are star players in making a fine bone broth. Often people are reluctant about these ingredients, unless they grew up in a different country, in which case I sometimes hear, "Yes, that's how we did it when I was growing up." Or even, "We used to eat the feet right off the bone; they are so delicious!" Even in many parts of Europe they still make use of every last animal part. It is now more important than ever for us to get back to traditional food preparation and honor the wisdom of our past. These inexpensive super foods are a must for the GAPS Diet.

Homemade Chicken Broth
Makes about 4 quarts

When we make chicken broth we make it in one of three ways: using a whole stewing hen or layer; with the carcasses from a roasted chicken or two; or with 3 to 4 pounds of necks, backs, and wings (or a combination). With a roasted chicken, we often save the carcass in the freezer until we have enough to make broth.

1 3- to 4-pound stewing hen, 1–2 chicken carcasses, or 3–4 pounds chicken necks, backs, and wings
4 quarts filtered water
2–4 chicken feet (optional)
1–2 chicken heads (optional)
2 tablespoons apple cider vinegar
3 celery stalks, coarsely chopped
2 carrots, coarsely chopped
1 onion, quartered
Handful of fresh parsley
Sea salt

Put the chicken or carcasses in a pot with 4 quarts of water; add the chicken feet and heads (if you're using them) and the vinegar. Let sit for 30 minutes, to give the vinegar time to leach the minerals out of the bones. Add the vegetables and turn on the heat. Bring to a boil and skim the scum. Reduce to barely a simmer, cover, and cook for 6 to 24 hours. During the last 10 minutes of cooking, throw in a handful of fresh parsley for added flavor and minerals. Let the broth cool, strain it, and take any remaining meat off the bones to use in future cooking. Add sea salt to taste and drink the broth as is or store it in the fridge (up to 5 to 7 days), or freezer (up to 6 months), for use in soups and stews.

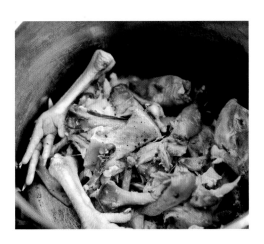
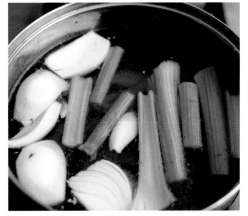
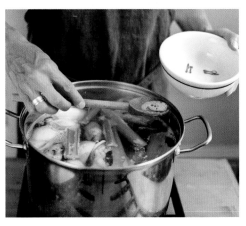
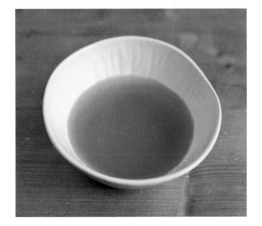

Beef Broth
Makes about 4 quarts

It's important to include both marrow and knuckle bones so you will reap the benefits of both gelatin and marrow. Broths can be cooked over time, so if you want to turn it off at night you can resume cooking in the morning. Just bring to a boil, skim the scum off the top, and discard.

Some people roast bones in the oven for 15 to 30 minutes before throwing them in the pot to improve the flavor of the stock, but Dr. Campbell-McBride advises using raw bones.

3–4 pounds beef marrow and
   knuckle bones
2 pounds meaty bones, such as short ribs
½ cup raw apple cider vinegar
4 quarts filtered water

3 celery stalks, halved
3 carrots, halved
3 onions, quartered
Handful of fresh parsley
Sea salt

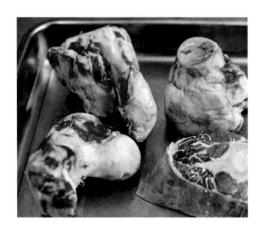
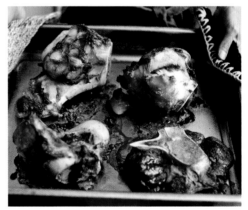
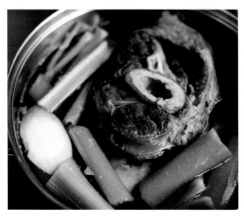
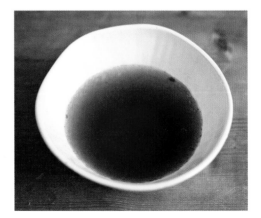

Place the bones in a pot, add the apple cider vinegar and water, and let the mixture sit for 1 hour so the vinegar can leach the minerals out of the bones. (Add more water if needed to cover the bones.) Add the vegetables, bring to a boil, and skim the scum from the top and discard. Reduce to a low simmer, cover, and cook for 24 to 72 hours. During the last 10 minutes of cooking, throw in a handful of fresh parsley for added flavor and minerals. Let the broth cool and strain it, making sure all the marrow is knocked out of the marrow bones and into the broth. Add sea salt to taste and drink the broth as is or store it in the fridge (up to 5 to 7 days) or freezer (up to 6 months) for use in soups and stews.

Fish Broth
Serves 4 to 6

2 pounds whole fresh non-oily fish heads and bones such as cod, sole, halibut, rockfish, whiting, flounder, or snapper (heads alone make a delicious stock)

¼ cup raw apple cider vinegar
About 2 quarts filtered water
Handful of fresh parsley
Sea salt

Place the fish heads and bones in a stockpot. Add the vinegar and cover with water. Bring to a simmer and skim the scum. Simmer for 4 to 24 hours. During the last 10 minutes of cooking throw in a handful of fresh parsley for added flavor and minerals. Let cool and strain. Add salt to taste and drink the broth as is or store it in the fridge (up to 5 to 7 days) or freezer (up to 6 months) for use in soups and stew.

To Keep or Not to Keep?
When Broth (or Stock) Goes Bad

People often call me or email me to ask about their broth. *Has it gone bad? How long does it stay good in the fridge? How long can it stay at room temperature? How do I know when to chuck it?*

Well, here is the long and short of it, according to GAPS chef Monica Corrado. If your broth is sealed with a layer of fat, then you are good to go for about six months! If the broth is exposed to air, on the other hand, it is good in the fridge for five to seven days. In this case, when you take it out, bring it to a boil, skim the scum—and you will have another week to use it. If you ever find it smells off, toss it out. Likewise, if you bring it to a boil and the scum keeps coming and coming—again, it's time to throw it out! If you stick to these rules, you will do just fine.

Nuts and Seeds

Sally Fallon Morell explains in her book *Nourishing Traditions* that nuts and seeds are best when soaked and dehydrated. She calls them "crispy nuts." All nuts, grains, beans, and seeds have phytic acid and enzyme inhibitors otherwise known as "anti-nutrients." A diet heavy in these anti-nutrients can cause digestive irritation as well as nutrient deficiencies. Phytic acid binds to minerals and blocks the absorption of many key nutrients in the body. Enzyme inhibitors bind to enzymes and decrease their activity. Enzyme inhibitors and phytates are nature's defense mechanism protecting nuts, seeds, grains, and legumes, allowing them to survive until they are in their optimal sprouting conditions and can become a plant. When we soak nuts and seeds, we are essentially creating the optimal moist environment that nature intended, and allowing them to germinate. Starting this germination process and neutralizing the enzyme inhibitors and phytic acid

The Critical Place of Healthy Fats in the GAPS Diet

Healthy fats are one of the pillars of the GAPS Diet. Without the proper fats, you will not last long on the diet. The fats are where it's at! As a former fat-free girl, let me tell you that fat does not make you fat. Fat is in fact what satiates you, keeps your blood sugar stable, and helps to heal the gut lining. Dr. Natasha Campbell-McBride tells us to eat "natural fats in their natural state," and that the most important fats for those on the GAPS Diet are animal fats (*Gut and Psychology Syndrome*, Revised and Expanded Edition, page 275).

The healthiest fats are pork lard, beef tallow, duck fat, goose fat, shmaltz (chicken fat), olive oil, coconut oil, ghee, palm oil, and butter. You will also get fat from your home-made stocks since bone marrow contains fat-soluble nutrients such as vitamins A, D, and E. Fatty acids provide essential raw minerals to aid and rebuild the gut lining.

Make sure to mix it up so you are getting different fatty acid profiles all the time. But avoid all saturated vegetable fats and trans-fats; these are *not* healthy fats and are actually quite damaging to the body.

When you add fats to your broth or stock, you are helping your body assimilate the nutrients. Feel free to add a tablespoon or two of animal fat, coconut oil, ghee, or cultured cream to every bowl of soup! When I call for you to add "good-quality animal fat" to any of the recipes in this book, you choose! I will give you a suggested fat, but feel free to substitute what you have or go by the flavor you desire (coconut oil or ghee may be more desirable in a sweet dessert, for instance, whereas lard and tallow may pair better with savory meats and roasted vegetables). As long as you stick to the "healthy fats" mentioned above, it's your call.

makes them easier on our digestive systems and allows us to better absorb the nutrients. Traditional cultures went to great lengths to make their nuts, seeds, grains, and legumes more digestible. See resources for information about bulk-ordering nuts. Be careful—they're addictive!

Sprouted Seeds

Place ½ to 1 cup raw seeds in a clean quart-sized mason jar, and cover 2 inches above the top with filtered water. Cover the jar with cheesecloth and a rubber band, and let it sit overnight for 10 hours in a cool place. Drain the seeds, rinse, and drain again; replace the cheesecloth, then invert the jar and position it at an angle in a Pyrex measuring cup or bowl. This will allow air to circulate and water to continue draining. Rinse the seeds every 12 hours, and repeat the process until sprouting begins—about 2 days. Dump the sprouted seeds onto a plate or cookie sheet, and let them dry completely. Then put them back into a clean, dry jar, cap it, and store in the fridge.

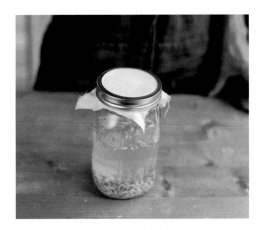
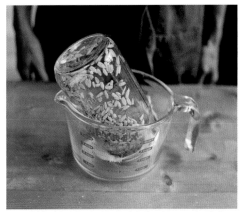
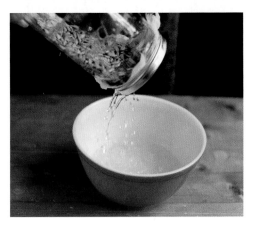
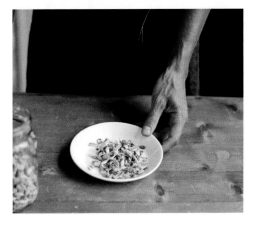

Crispy Nuts

Place 4 cups raw nuts in a large jar or glass bowl. Cover with warm filtered water. Gently stir in some sea salt (use the measuring table). Soak for 7 hours. Strain, rinse, and place in a dehydrator or oven at no more than 150°F for 24 hours, or until crisp. Store all nuts in an airtight container in the fridge or freezer for up to 6 months.

Note: *Cashews are not truly raw since they're heated to 350°F while still in their shell to neutralize a toxic oil called cardol before they go to market. Therefore, it's not necessary to dehydrate them after soaking, but roasting will make them the tastiest. Follow the regular soaking instructions (soak for no longer than 6 hours), then spread them out on a cookie sheet. Roast in the oven at 200 to 250°F for 12 hours for optimal flavor and crunch.*

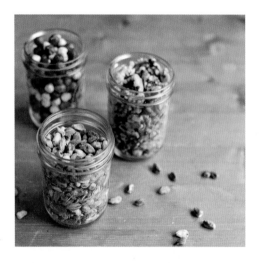
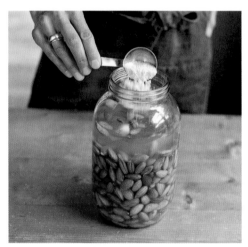
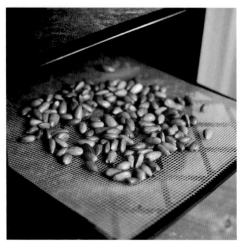
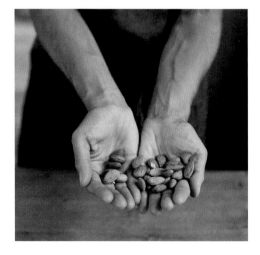

Salt measurements for soaking nuts (4 cups nuts):

Pecans	2 teaspoons	Hazelnuts	1 tablespoon
Walnuts	2 teaspoons	Cashews	1 tablespoon
Peanuts	1 tablespoon	Pumpkin seeds	2 tablespoons
Pine nuts	1 tablespoon	Sunflower seeds	2 tablespoons
Almonds	1 tablespoon	Pistachios	No soaking required!
Macadamia nuts	1 tablespoon		

Nut Milk

In a blender or Vitamix, place 1 cup crispy nuts and 4 cups fresh filtered water. Blend for 30 seconds to a minute. Strain the milk into your pitcher through a sieve or nut milk bag. Gently press down on the solids or squeeze the bag to release all of the milk. Add spices or sweeteners as you wish. Store in the fridge for 2 to 3 days. See "Nut Pulp" (page 257) for several nut pulp recipes.

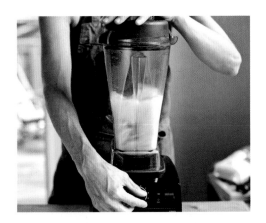
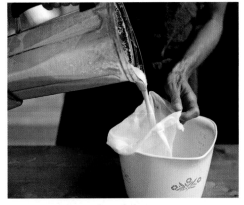
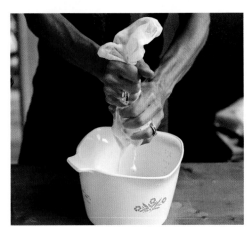
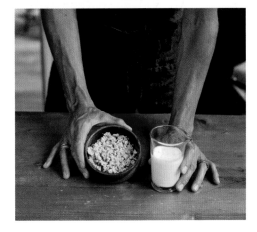

Nut Flour

Place 4 cups crispy nuts in a food processor or Vitamix. Process until a flour-like consistency is achieved. Watch carefully, as the mixture will quickly turn to nut butter if you let it go too long! Store in a dark airtight container in the fridge for up to 3 months, or freeze for up to 6 months.

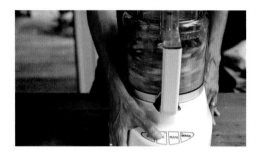
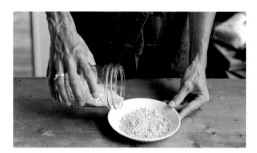

Nut Butter

Place 4 cups crispy nuts in your food processor. Blend for a good 5 minutes, scraping down the sides as necessary. Add a generous pinch of sea salt and about 1 to 2 tablespoons coconut oil. For a sweeter nut butter, add a tablespoon of raw honey. Scrape the nut butter into a jar, cap, and store in the fridge.

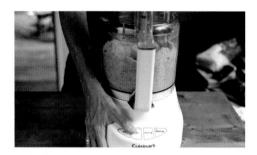
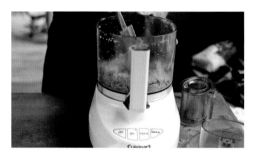
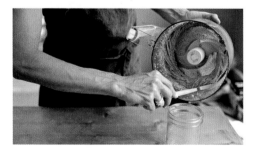
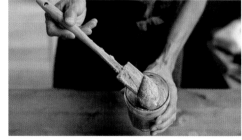

Nut Crackers

Place 2 cups sprouted and finely ground nuts in your food processor. Add ½ teaspoon salt, ¼ teaspoon garlic powder, 2 tablespoons fresh herbs (or 1 tablespoon dried), 1 to 2 tablespoons coconut oil, 1 egg (or 1 flax or chia egg; see the note below), and ½ cup raw Parmesan cheese (optional, on Full GAPS). Blend all the dry ingredients together; add in the wet ingredients and blend again. Mold into a ball and place in the fridge for 20 minutes.

Using a cutting board, or two pieces of parchment paper, roll out the dough to a thickness of ⅛ inch. Cut with a knife in your desired shapes. Place on a nonstick sheet in your dehydrator at 145°F for 12 hours. Flip and dehydrate for another 12 hours. If you don't have a dehydrator, place in your oven on the lowest setting for about 1 hour or until crisp, flipping halfway through. Store in an airtight container in the fridge.

Note: *To make a flax or chia egg, combine 1 tablespoon of ground flax or chia seeds with 3 tablespoons of water and let stand for 5 minutes.*

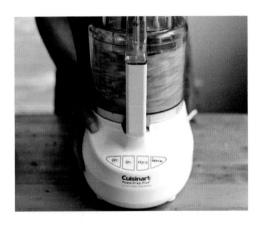
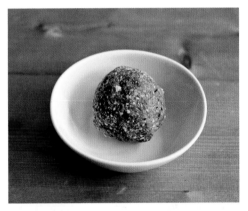
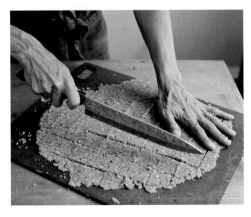
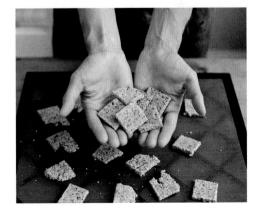

Coconut

Coconut to the rescue! For people who cannot tolerate dairy, coconut is a wonderful alternative. Coconut oil is made up of medium chain triglycerides and is an easily digested fat that supplies a quick boost of energy to the body. It's great for the brain and is also antiviral, antimicrobial, and antibacterial. For those with a dairy intolerance—as well as those without—this is a great alternative with loads of nutrients and delicious flavor to boot!

Opening a Young Thai Coconut

Scrape away the thick white husk until you see the coconut's rounded top. Using a cleaver or a heavy knife, strike swiftly and make four marks around the dome, creating a 2-inch square. As you keep striking these spots, the coconut will open up. Peel off the top, and pour the coconut water through a strainer to remove any bits of shell from your fresh coconut water. Use the back of a spoon to remove the young coconut meat; it will be more rubbery than that of a mature coconut. Use it in smoothies, or to make yogurt (recipe follows). The water can also be used in smoothies, or it can be popped in the fridge for a nice electrolyte drink. You can also ferment the coconut water and make a refreshing coconut water kefir using water kefir grains (see resources).

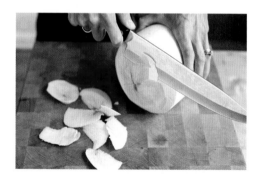
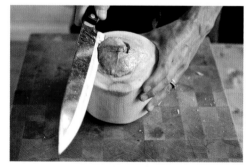
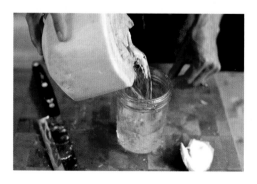
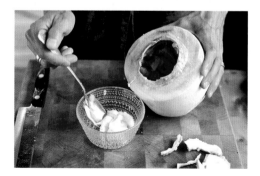

Coconut Milk

Rinse the meat from 1 young Thai coconut, making sure to discard all hard brown bits of shell, and toss it in the blender with 2 cups filtered water (or coconut water for a sweeter drink). Blend for a minute or so, strain through a cheesecloth, and enjoy! If you're using a mature coconut, use 1 cup meat with 3 cups water.

Variation: Coconut milk with dehydrated coconut flakes. Place 2½ cups just-boiled, filtered water in your blender (the hot water helps to release the fat from the flakes, making a thicker, better-tasting coconut milk). Add 1½ cups coconut flakes. Blend for a few minutes, then strain through a cheesecloth. Squeeze gently to get out all of the "milk." Store coconut milk in a glass jar in the fridge. Use coconut pulp to make coconut flour (recipe follows) or for yummy desserts such as Chocolate Truffles, Gingersnaps, or Macaroons (see "Nut Pulp," page 257).

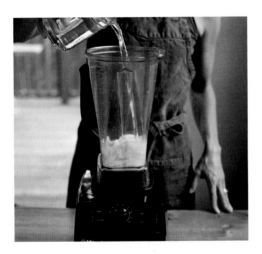
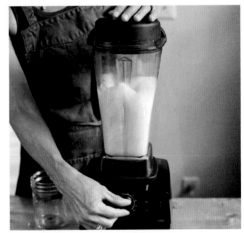

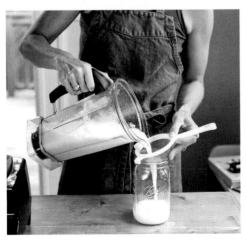
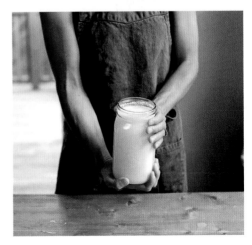

Coconut Butter

Pour 4 cups unsweetened coconut flakes into a food processor or high-speed blender. Start by pulsing, scraping down the sides with a spatula. This will take 10 to 20 minutes to process (a food processor is faster than a blender). Store in a glass jar in the cupboard. Add flavor if desired (see Coconut Bark, page 275).

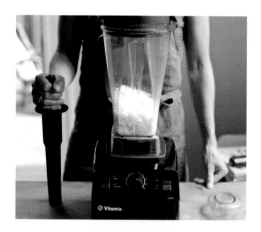
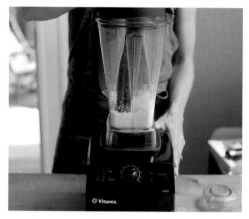
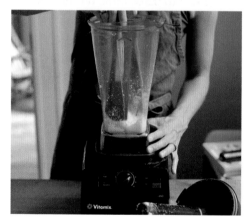
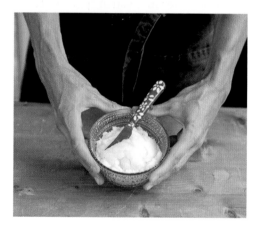

Coconut Milk Yogurt

Blend 2 cups of young Thai coconut meat with ¼ to ½ cup coconut water, water kefir, or filtered water until smooth and creamy. Pour through a strainer into a clean, quart-sized mason jar, filling it three-quarters of the way, allowing room for the yogurt to expand. Add two capsules probiotic powder, or ¼ teaspoon loose powder, and stir. Place the jar in a yogurt maker, oven (with the light on), or dehydrator at 110°F for 24 hours and up to 72 hours.

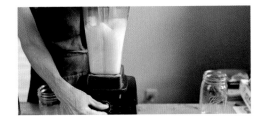
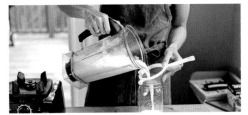
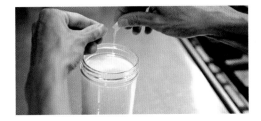
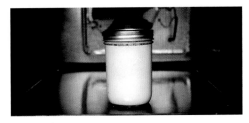

Coconut Milk Kefir

Add 1 package kefir starter, 2 tablespoons milk kefir grains, or ½ cup kefir from a previous batch to 4 cups homemade coconut milk and stir. Cap and leave on the counter in a warm spot for 24 to 36 hours (I like to place mine on the top of my turned-on dehydrator, especially in the winter months when my countertop isn't too warm). Shake a few times throughout the day. Strain the grains and start a new batch. Store kefir in the fridge. For additional information see "Raw Milk Kefir," page 28. (Note: Photos reflect smaller serving)

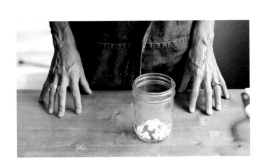
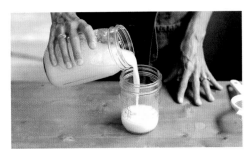
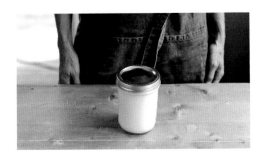
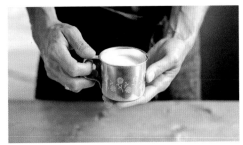

Coconut Flour

After straining your coconut milk, spread the pulp on a baking tray lined with parchment paper or a nonstick sheet in your dehydrator. Dry in the oven on the lowest temperature, or in your dehydrator on 90°F for about an hour, or until all the moisture has evaporated. Pour the dried coconut pulp into a high-powered blender or your Vitamix, and blend on high for 30 seconds until you have coconut flour. Store in an airtight jar. This will be considerably lighter and fluffier than what you buy in the store—not to mention healthier. Store-bought coconut flour is not allowed on the GAPS Diet because it's too high in fiber.

Note: *For a quicker method, you can also blend dried coconut flakes in a high-speed blender until they become flour. Just be careful not to let it go too long, or you'll end up with coconut butter.*

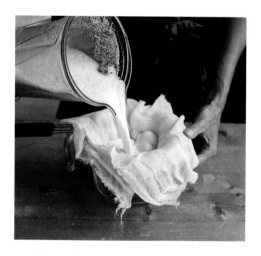 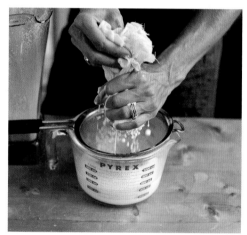

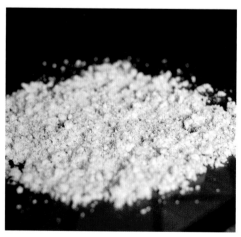 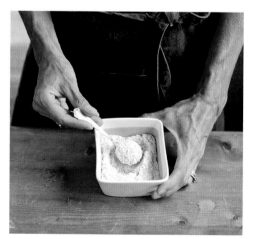

Raw Dairy

Raw dairy is filled with beneficial bacteria and is easily digested because its enzymes haven't been altered or destroyed by the high heat of pasteurization. If for some reason raw dairy is absolutely not available, you can substitute high-quality pasteurized organic whole milk from grass-fed cows. When you culture dairy into foods like kefir and yogurt, you will at least be adding back some of the beneficial bacteria that have been lost through pasteurization.

Raw-Milk Yogurt

To make raw-milk yogurt, it's best to find a trusted source of raw milk. If you're unable to find raw milk, you can still make yogurt with the very best-quality organic whole milk from grass-fed cows. Try to find lightly pasteurized, not ultrapasteurized or homogenized milk. Raw-milk yogurt tends to have a thinner consistency than yogurt from pasteurized milk. If you would like a thicker-consistency yogurt, you can strain it through cheesecloth and separate out some of the whey. You can then use the whey to culture vegetables, soak nut flours, or add to smoothies or juices for some extra probiotics. Goat's-milk yogurt is a great first option since it's often easier to digest; many people on GAPS tolerate this better. If you cannot find goat's milk, go ahead with raw cow's milk and see how you do.

If you're using raw milk, it's preferable not to heat it; otherwise you might destroy its molecular structure. Instead, just place raw milk into a quart-sized mason jar and add 1 tablespoon starter culture (yogurt) per cup of milk. Stir gently to incorporate; cap and place in a dehydrator at 110°F or in your oven with the light on for 24 hours or longer (with a reminder sticky note on the oven door). Monica Corrado recommends finding a very good-quality stainless-steel thermos and heating it with hot water before adding raw milk and starter. Cap and leave on the counter for 24 hours. The thermos will keep it at 110°F for 24 hours. After 24 hours, place the yogurt in the fridge and cool.

If you are using pasteurized dairy, place 1 quart milk into a pot over low heat, and attach a thermometer. Heat the milk to 180°F. Remove from the heat and cool to 110°F (about 10 minutes). Place ¼ cup of starter yogurt in a quart-sized mason jar. Carefully add the heated milk up to the shoulder of the jar (about 1 inch from the top). Stir gently to incorporate; cap and place in a dehydrator at 110°F (it needs 110°F for 24 hours to ensure that the lactose is fully digested) or in your oven with the light on for 24 hours (with a reminder sticky note on the oven door).

After 24 hours, place the yogurt in the fridge and cool. You will notice that the cream separates to the top. Just give it a big stir before serving—or enjoy a little cream. It is delicious and so healing for the gut!

Making your own yogurt is a huge money saver. I make 8 quarts of yogurt for $20 since I pay $10 per gallon for my raw milk. You might be able to find your raw milk for as low as $7 per gallon. To buy 8 quarts of organic yogurt at the grocery store would cost me about $60, not to mention the time traveled to get there and the waste of eight plastic containers.

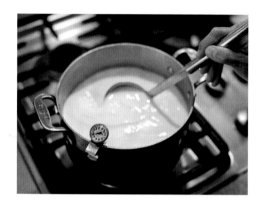
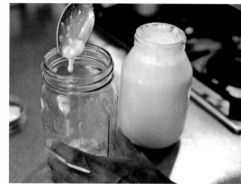
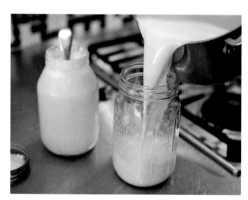
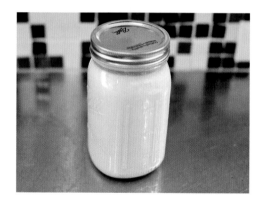

Raw-Milk Kefir

Making kefir is very easy, and it is so nutritious. The lactic acid produced in the fermentation process is very soothing for the gut. Kefir is an excellent source for B vitamins, vitamin K, and biotin. Kefir provides us with many additional strains of probiotics beyond what yogurt can supply. Kefir grains are rubbery, look like little gummy bears, and often vary in their size and shape. They are safe to eat if one escapes through your strainer. Kefir is an excellent option for salad dressings or as a substitute for milk, buttermilk, yogurt, or sour cream. I often use kefir to soak store-bought almond flour if I'm not making my own from soaked and dehydrated nuts.

Place your kefir grains, starter (see resources), or ½ cup kefir from a previous batch in a clean, quart-sized mason jar. Fill the jar to the shoulder with room-temperature, fresh, raw milk, cap, and leave on the counter for 24 hours—longer if you like a more sour taste. (I like to leave mine on top of my warm dehydrator.) Gently shake the kefir a few times throughout the fermentation process to make sure all the milk is being fermented. When the milk is finished fermenting, you can either pop it directly in the fridge or strain and start a new batch immediately. I have about four batches of kefir going at a time, so I just keep them in the fridge with the grains and rotate as needed.

When I'm making a new batch of kefir, I use about ½ cup of my existing kefir as a starter for the next batch.

If you're using pasteurized milk, heat the milk to 180°F and allow it to cool to 110°F before adding the starter. Follow the instructions above.

Kefir can be quite sour or effervescent, so it may take a little doctoring for kids to really enjoy the taste, especially if they're used to the sugary store-bought kefirs. I recommend starting your children with it unsweetened early on, so they develop a taste for its natural sweetness. We enjoy kefir with a little raw honey, coconut shreds, ground flax seeds, some crispy nuts, and fresh fruit. Another great idea is to do a second fermentation. Just strain your fresh-made kefir into another mason jar, add fresh fruit, cap, and leave it on the counter for an additional 24 hours.

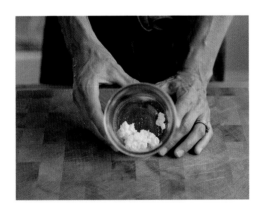
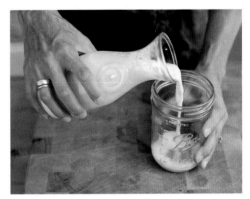
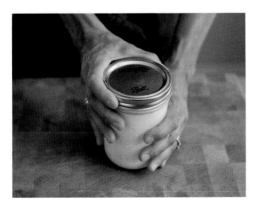
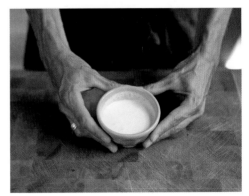

Homemade Cultured Cream or Sour Cream

Place slightly less than 1 quart raw cream in a quart-sized mason jar. Inoculate with ½ cup of your starter (either store-bought crème fraîche, sour cream, yogurt, kefir, a previous batch of cultured cream, or 1 packet of yogurt or kefir starter). Cap and let sit in a warm spot for at least 24 hours; it might take up to 48 hours to properly thicken. This is delicious with honey and cinnamon or garlic and herbs (fresh herbs in Stage 2 and dried herbs in Stage 5). And it's a perfect way to add some great fats and live cultures to any smoothie, soup, or Mexican dish. (Photos reflect a smaller serving)

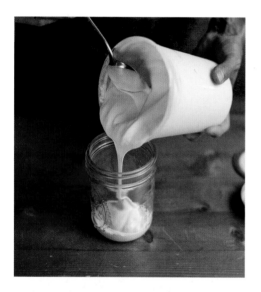
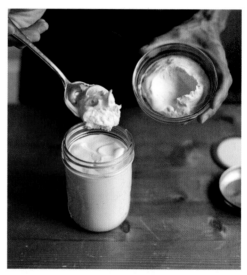
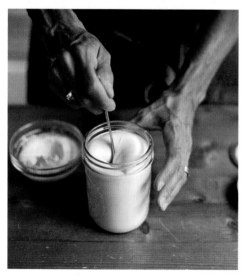
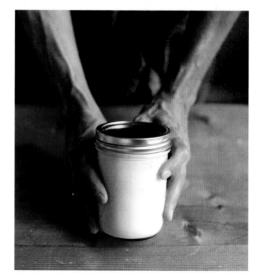

Fresh Cultured Butter

Place 1 quart fresh cultured cream into a food processor or standing mixer fitted with the whisk attachment. Beat on medium-high until the cream starts to turn yellow as it separates from the buttermilk. In about 2 minutes, you will have a ball of butter. Turn the machine off, pour out the buttermilk, and briefly beat again. Repeat the process until all the remaining buttermilk is really strained out, then place the ball in a bowl and press out the last of the buttermilk. Rinse the butter under cool water, pat it dry with a paper towel, add sea salt if desired, and store it in a crock in the fridge.

Another fun way to make butter, especially with kids, is to shake it yourself. My kids all did this in preschool. If you place a pint of cream in a quart-sized mason jar, cap the jar, and start shaking, you will rather quickly see it turn to butter. Remove from the jar and pour off the buttermilk. Run the butter under cool water to remove the last drips of buttermilk.

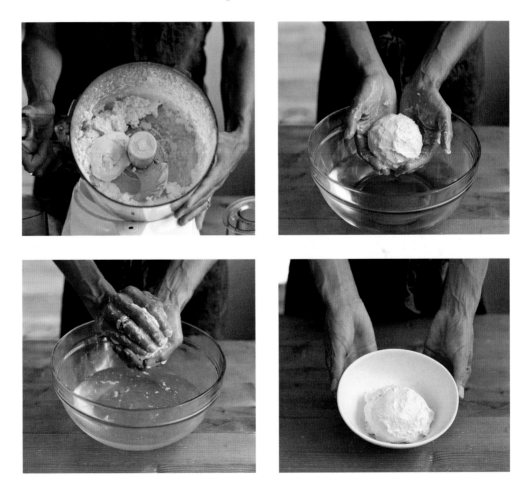

Ghee

Ghee is a wonderful fat for cooking because it has a higher smoke point (485°F) than most oils, so it's great for sautéing, pan-frying, and roasting at higher temps. It's not as hard as you may think to make your own ghee.

Place 1 cup butter in a medium-sized, heavy-bottomed saucepan and melt over low heat, or put it in a pan in the oven at 200°F. Simmer until the butter clarifies (it should be foamy on top and clear butter underneath)—about 10 minutes, or until the butter stops crackling. Let the ghee cool for 20 minutes, then carefully skim any foam from the top with a fine-mesh skimmer or a large spoon, and strain it into a jar or crock through a double layer of cheesecloth. Store in an airtight container in the cabinet or fridge. Ghee does not need to be refrigerated.

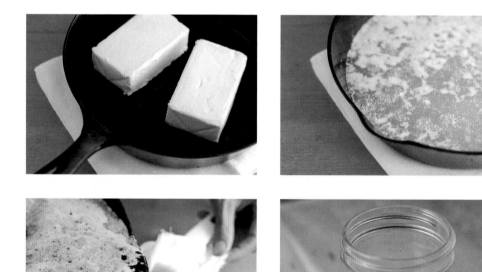

Yogurt or Kefir Cheese

Place cheesecloth, or a tea towel, in a strainer over a glass bowl and pour in 1 quart fresh raw-milk yogurt or kefir. Cover with a plate or towel, and leave on the counter or refrigerate overnight. You may also hang the tea towel or cheesecloth from a cabinet knob with a rubber band and allow it to drip into a bowl set below overnight. Remove the cheese from the cheesecloth and strainer, and shape it into a ball.

The clear yellow liquid that is the by-product of straining the cheese is called whey. Reserve the whey for use in smoothies, soups, and juices; as a starter to inoculate your cultured vegetables; or to soak your nut flours. Whey is an excellent source of healthy bacteria, and it's great for the gut when tolerated.

You can add whatever you want to the cheese. Here are a few ideas to get you started:

- Fold in chopped garlic, fresh thyme, and rosemary with a pinch of salt and a generous drizzle of olive oil on top.
- Fold in a tablespoon of honey, a teaspoon of vanilla, a pinch of cinnamon, and a pinch of salt for a sweet frosting or cheese.
- Yogurt and kefir cheese have become staples in our house. With homemade crackers, there really is no better!

Note: *Fresh herbs are not allowed until Stage 2, and dried spices are not allowed until Stage 5 of the Introduction Diet.*

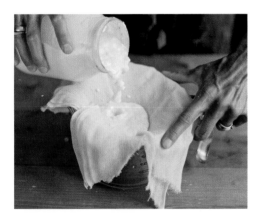
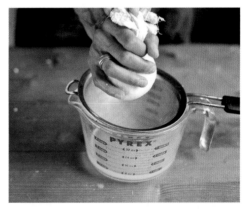
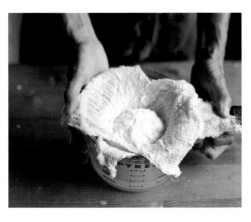
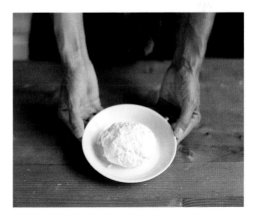

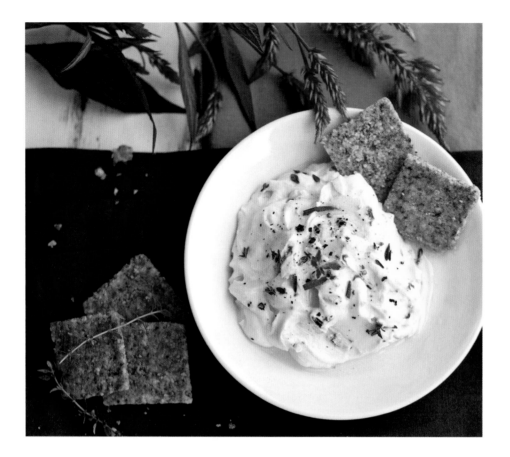

Dairy Sensitivity Test

If you have digestive disorders or food intolerances, Dr. Campbell-McBride recommends starting with the GAPS Introduction Diet, which calls for initial abstinence from dairy. This will help your gut lining heal faster than it will on the Full GAPS diet; thus you might be able to handle some well-fermented raw dairy after the Intro's initial stages. However, before reintroducing dairy to your diet, it is important to do the sensitivity test. (See *Gut and Psychology Syndrome*, Revised and Expanded Edition, page 120, for details).

At night, place a small dab of the food in question on the inside of your wrist. You may have to blend it with a little water if it's a solid or dry good. Let it dry and leave on for the remainder of the night. In the morning check to see if there is any irritation to the skin. If so, then avoid the food for another few weeks and repeat the sensitivity test. If there is no irritation, then you can slowly introduce the food to your diet. Start with 1 teaspoon per day for three to five days. Follow along with instructions from once again, my hero, GAPS chef Monica Corrado: Bear in mind that medical conditions more complicated than a basic dairy sensitivity may require diagnosis via in-depth clinical testing, such as blood work.

Introducing Dairy
Monica Corrado, MA, CNC, traditional food and GAPS chef

If you have no sensitivity to dairy, you can start with any kind of dairy on the Introduction Diet: whey, yogurt, cultured cream, and kefir. (There is no cheese allowed on the Introduction Diet.) For those with known dairy allergies, those who have shown an allergy to dairy products on the skin sensitivity test, or those who are on Full GAPS but did not do the Intro Diet, here is the protocol for introducing dairy. For additional information, refer to "What About Dairy?" and "Dairy Introduction Structure" in *Gut and Psychology Syndrome*, Revised and Expanded Edition by Dr. Campbell-McBride (pages 119–27).

1. Begin with homemade ghee or a ghee free of preservatives and other additives. Ghee is pure milk fat. It contains no lactose or casein.

2. If ghee is tolerated, six weeks later introduce organic butter (preferably unsalted or with sea salt). Organic butter is pure milk fat and a little whey. (Whey is a milk protein, which is easier to digest than casein.)

3. If butter is tolerated, six to twelve weeks later introduce homemade sour cream (crème fraîche) made with full-fat raw cow's cream. Homemade sour cream is mostly milk fat. It contains some milk protein, but no lactose if cultured for twenty-four hours. Culture the cream with yogurt and start by eating 1 teaspoon per day; increase to 1 to 2 cups per day. Introduce also homemade yogurt made from full-fat raw cow's or goat's milk. Be sure to culture the milk for twenty-four hours to predigest the lactose. Start with 1 teaspoon per day and increase to 1 to 2 cups per day.

4. If yogurt and sour cream are tolerated, six to twelve weeks later introduce homemade kefir made from full-fat raw cow's or goat's milk, and raw cream cultured with kefir for twenty-four hours. Start with 1 teaspoon per day and gradually increase the amount until you are having 1 to 2 cups per day.

5. Introduce cheese (start with cheddar and Parmesan) by eating a mouthful with a meal and checking for a reaction after three to five days. If there is none, then continue with cheese. Cheeses allowed on the Full GAPS Diet (organic and raw-milk are preferred) include Romano, Havarti, Roquefort, Swiss, Stilton, Muenster, blue cheese, brick cheese, Brie, Parmesan, cheddar, Colby, Limburger, Gorgonzola, cottage cheese, Gouda, Edam, Asiago, and Camembert.

6. After about two years on the diet, try some commercially produced, full-fat, live, organic yogurt, sour cream, and crème fraîche.

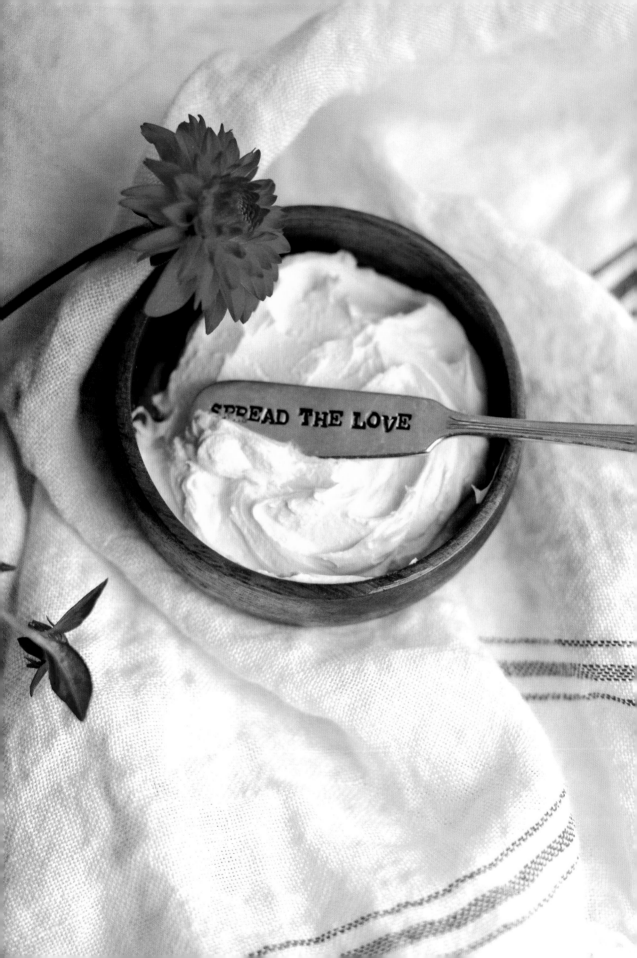

The GAPS Introduction Diet

The GAPS Introduction Diet is a very healing protocol that will restore the balance between the good and the bad bacteria in your gut, so that you can regain and take control of your health. But it is not meant to be a long phase. Although the Full GAPS Diet is most often a minimum two-year commitment, the GAPS Intro Diet typically lasts anywhere from eighteen to 30 days, roughly 3 to 5 days per stage. There is no harm in staying on the Introduction Diet for longer periods of time as long as you are eating plenty of quality animal protein, fats, and freshly pressed juices. My husband and I completed a month of the Intro Diet before going back and repeating it with our children. (We also started them on the first day of school vacation, so we knew we had ten days for them to adjust.) Before you embark on the intro diet, please read *Gut and Psychology Syndrome*, Revised and Expanded Edition (pages 142–52) by Dr. Natasha Campbell-McBride.

If you are new to this way of eating, or new to cooking from scratch, consider starting with a couple of weeks, or even months, on the Full GAPS Diet in order to get your feet wet and get used to your new normal in regard to the foods you'll be eating and how they need to be prepared, before you start the Intro Diet. People often feel better right away, simply by eliminating processed foods and eating the Full GAPS Diet. Then you can return to the GAPS Intro Diet with more confidence in the kitchen (and in the grocery store). But to truly heal the gut, when you are ready, you need to go back to the beginning and follow the GAPS Intro Diet Protocol.

There is no question we were nervous as the day approached that we'd start our five kids on the GAPS Intro Diet. Three nine-year-olds, a six-year-old, and a five-year-old: How in the world was it all going to go? Well, there were struggles, of course, but I must say it went much better than I'd ever dreamed. In fact, I think the hardest part was just deciding to do it: picking a date and actually starting. My husband was a total hero those first few days when our kids came down to soup for breakfast. As he showed me, courage, strong will, and a no-nonsense attitude are key. Over their initial sniffly tears, upset stomachs, and whiny complaints, Nick simply stated, "It's soup or nothin', no two ways about it." I stood there in the background, so grateful that I had his strength, support, and good humor for the road ahead of us.

The point at which you move from one stage to the next is your call. We did five days at each stage, but you may bust through them at two days a pop. Likewise, you might need to hang out at a certain stage for a few weeks. If you are symptom-free and things are feeling right, move on to the next stage. If any adverse reactions occur with the reintroduction of new foods (for example, more trips to the bathroom, bloating, hand flapping, or hyperactivity), you will know that you moved ahead too quickly. No worries. Simply return to the previous stage for at least two to five days, and allow for more healing to take place before trying again. Respect your bio-individuality and move forward, or backward, accordingly.

Once you're in a groove, it moves along quickly. Before you know it, you will be on to the next stage! We made it a kind of game, and the kids got excited about counting down days to the next stage. It might sound a little desperate, but you do what you have to do to get through. Screen time, little presents, an extra book before bed, or some new Legos didn't hurt, either. Kids on GAPS are real troopers and deserve encouragement. Keep in mind that this is a big transition for your family—a little treat here and there goes a long way. Stay with it, stay strong, and follow through! Likewise, if you are an adult going through this without kids: Please, pamper yourself! Take a day off and curl up in bed with a good book or TV show. Or have a nap, then go to the movies with some friends. Cut yourself some slack in these first few weeks, pat yourself on the back, and take whatever you can off your plate!

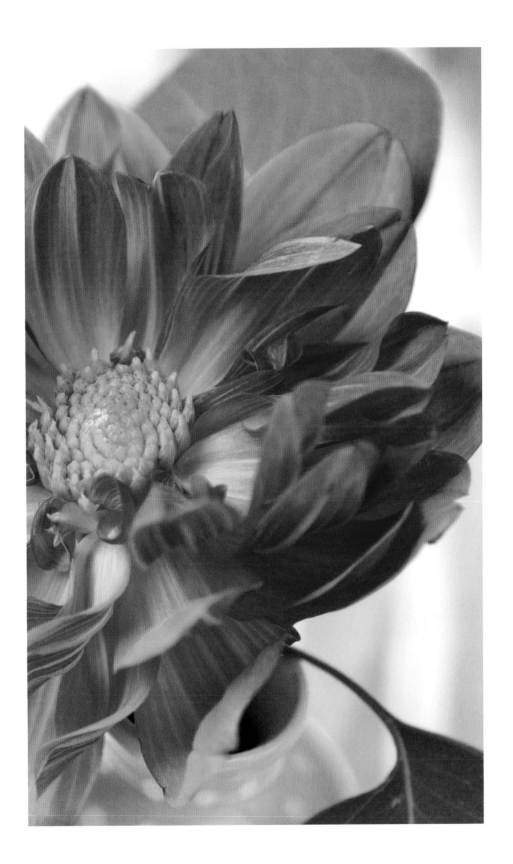

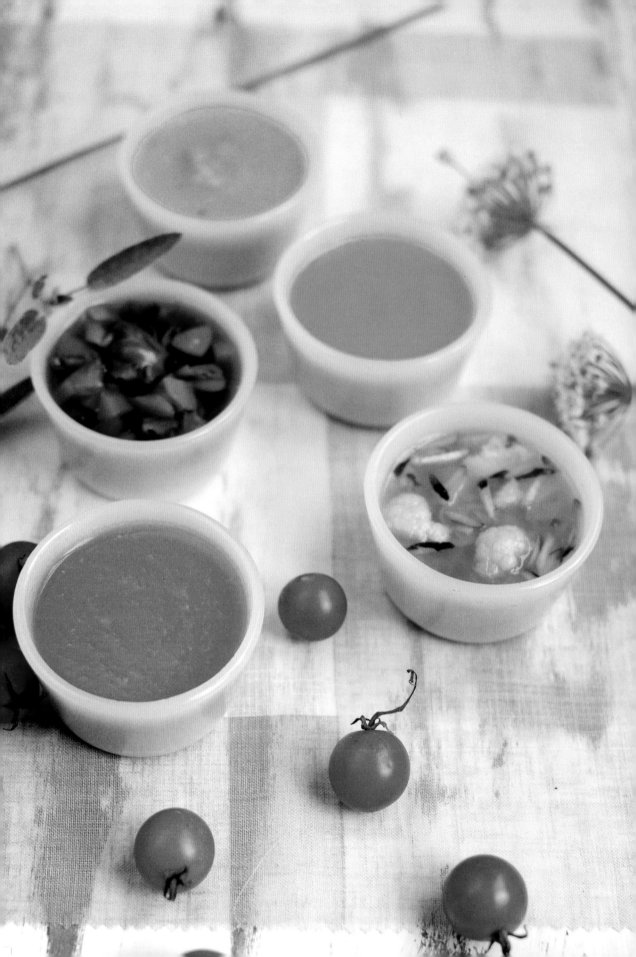

Stage 1

Okay, here we go! You now have the knowledge and desire to move forward with the GAPS Diet. So here is the nitty-gritty, down-and-dirty truth about what you can expect for the next month or so. In a word, it's all about soup.

Soup, when properly prepared from nutrient-dense meat stock, provides an exceptionally easy-to-digest and nourishing meal that begins to heal the gut wall. The proteins in meat stock are partially broken down, giving your body a chance to rest while reaping the benefits of the stock's healing power. Having these soups also removes most fiber from your diet, again allowing your digestive tract time to heal. Although you will have options for what kind of soup, just know that you will be eating what seems like dinner for breakfast and lunch for dinner. You will basically be throwing out all the food rules you are used to. Some days, you may even choose to have the same exact thing for breakfast, lunch, and dinner if menu planning feels like too much work!

On that note, always keep some soups on hand in the freezer in the event that cookin' just ain't gonna happen. I suggest making big batches of any three soups that are listed in this section, then simply alternating for the first several days. If you can prep them before officially starting the diet, you'll be psyched! My family mostly ate Basic Chicken Soup, Butternut Squash Soup, and Crock-Pot Beef Soup.

In between or after meals, we enjoyed a coconut cream as a treat, or a small spoonful of honey. (This was key in getting the kids to eat. If they knew they would get a little honey after finishing a meal, it was eaten up for sure.) Nick and I also had lots of ginger and turmeric tea with coconut oil and honey throughout the day. And try this boost with a probiotic bonus for the kids: Using a plastic, calibrated syringe, measure out 1 tablespoon of fermented pickle juice and take it orally three times a day. Eventually, you may work up to five "shots" a day per meal. All these little snacks, sips, and squirts will keep your blood sugar stable so that you're not crashing in between meals.

When you start Stage 1, bad bacteria begins to die off right away. It's possible that this will make you feel physically sick (nausea, exhaustion, runs to the bathroom, and so on). This, too, shall pass! For our family, it lasted only the first twenty-four hours, but every person has a different bacterial composition, and states of gut health vary as well. So the degree of die-off and discomfort will depend on the individual. No matter what, just stick with it, and keep thinking about how much better you'll feel on the other side of withdrawal. Remember, you are starving off those pesky, sugar-addicted bugs in your gut. They are pissed and hanging on for dear life. But if you can hold out and stick with the soup, your body will inevitably purge them by whatever means necessary.

Foods Allowed During Stage 1

Stage 1 is based on three components: stock and soups made with meats, fish, and vegetables; probiotic foods; and fats. When making your stock, be sure to use pastured meats and simmer only for a few hours to start out. Start every day with a glass of mineral or filtered water with fresh lemon juice.

In Stage 1, you can have:
- **Homemade stocks** from fish, beef, chicken, turkey, and lamb: Make sure to reserve and utilize bone marrow and soft tissues in soups
- **Soups** with well-boiled vegetables and meats
- **Meats:** beef, pork, lamb, goose, pheasant, turkey, shellfish, and chicken, boiled in stock or filtered water
- **Chopped liver:** Liver is a nutritional powerhouse that can be cooked into any soup
- **Well-cooked vegetables,** with all fibrous stems and peels removed: beets, bok choy, broccoli (no stalks), brussels sprouts, carrots, cauliflower (no stalks), collard greens, eggplant, French artichokes, garlic, green beans, kale, onions, peas, peppers, pumpkin, spinach, squash (winter and summer), tomatoes, turnips, and watercress
- **Animal fats:** tallow, lard, goose, chicken, duck
- **Coconut oil**
- **Sea salt**
- **Peppercorns:** black, green, and white (whole, to flavor soups and stocks only)
- **Probiotic foods:** 1 to 2 teaspoons per day of homemade fermented vegetable juices (pickle or sauerkraut) and whey, yogurt, sour cream/cultured cream, and kefir, cultured for at least twenty-four hours (see "Raw Dairy," page 27), if there is no dairy allergy; if you are sensitive to dairy, follow the dairy introduction protocol (page 35)
- **Filtered water**
- **Teas:** Fresh gingerroot and turmeric tea, and loose herbal tea (chamomile is good)
- **Lemon juice** mixed with warm filtered water
- **Raw honey** in small amounts

Making Soups During Stage 1

Vegetables

During the early stages of GAPS Intro Diet (Stage 1 through 3), soups are made by cooking vegetables in stock. When you move to Stage 4 and beyond, you can move to sautéing vegetables in healthy fat and then adding stock to make soup.

Fermented Foods

Fermented foods are essential to healing the gut and must be introduced right from the start. If you can handle dairy, add whey, yogurt, or sour cream to every bowl of soup. If you cannot handle dairy, be sure to add fermented vegetable juice to every bowl of soup. When you add homemade yogurt or cultured cream, the fat will help you to absorb all the nutrients in the soup. Be sure the temperature of the soup isn't too hot, since that will destroy the precious beneficial probiotic bacteria in the yogurt, cream, and fermented vegetable juices. Cultured cream is a wonderful addition to any soup: It provides not only a probiotic punch but also a healthy dose of fat-soluble vitamins. Vitamins A, D, E, and K are hard to get in modern diets, and they are essential to a healthy body. Raw cultured cream is a great source of vitamin A, and good healthy animal fats are the best way to nourish your body with the fat-soluble vitamins it needs!

Herbs and Spices

Fresh herbs are not allowed until Stage 2. However, with a "bouquet garni," the herbs infuse the soup and are not actually ingested, so feel free to use them to add flavor to any soup. A bouquet garni is a bundle of herbs tied together with cooking string, or wrapped in a bundle of cheesecloth and tied up with string. They are used to flavor soups, stocks, or stews. You can really put whichever herbs you desire in the bunch, but I most often tie together parsley, rosemary, thyme, bay leaf, and garlic. Fresh herbs are allowed in Stage 2 (and may be dried or fresh); spices (which should be ground) are not allowed until Stage 5. Pepper is a spice, so don't add it until Stage 5, although peppercorns are allowed in Stage 1; use them to flavor meat stock and then discard.

Once you have reached Stage 5, be sure to add sea salt and fresh cracked pepper to all of the Intro recipes! Speaking of sea salt, buy unrefined sea salt with a tinge of color. If it is white-white, it means it has been refined and stripped of many of the beneficial trace minerals that you want! See resources for good options.

Storage

If you ever have excess greens in your fridge, blanching and freezing is the answer. To blanch your greens, first remove the stems and discard them—they are too fibrous. Chop greens into 2-inch pieces. Place these in a pot of boiling water for 30 seconds, then remove and put in a bowl of ice water to stop the cooking process. Pat dry and store in single servings, in ziplock bags, in the freezer. When it's time to make soup, throw these right in your Crock-Pot or soup pot still frozen.

Helpful Definitions

Soup: Mostly liquid with a little bit of meat and vegetables
Stew: Half stock, half meat and vegetables
Casserole: Mostly meat and vegetables with a little bit of stock

Poached Chicken
Serves 6 to 8

This is a staple in our house because it is easy, quick, and delicious.

1 3- to 4-pound whole, organic, pastured chicken
2–3 celery stalks, chopped
1 onion, quartered
2 carrots, peeled and diced
4 quarts filtered water, or a little more if needed to cover the chicken
2 cloves garlic, peeled and crushed
1 tablespoon peppercorns
2 bay leaves
A few sprigs of fresh thyme, rosemary, or other herbs
Juice of one lemon
1 tablespoon unrefined sea salt

Remove the giblets from your chicken, rinse it with cold water, and pat it dry. Place the chicken in a large stockpot. Add the celery, onion, and carrots to the pot. Cover with filtered water, and add the garlic, peppercorns, bay leaves, fresh herbs, lemon juice, and a good pinch of sea salt. Bring the water to a boil, skim any scum from the top, and reduce the heat to a simmer for about an hour and 20 minutes. Remove the chicken and place it on a platter to cool for 20 minutes. Pull all the chicken off the bone and shred or dice for storage in Tupperware to use in various recipes throughout the week. Place the carcass back in the pot to make broth (page 12), or freeze the carcass for later use once on the Full GAPS diet.

Basic Chicken Soup
Serves 6 to 8

When we first started the GAPS Intro Diet, I remember making this soup and adding to it whatever vegetables I could find in my fridge. I was so hungry for nutrients that I could not get enough into my soups. Try cutting up zucchini and summer squash, turnips, or rutabaga. Throw in some fresh spinach. Get creative and add what you like. For my kids, I keep the basic recipe pretty simple since they each have their favorite add-ins. Some of the vegetables don't take long to cook (like spinach), so you can put them in at the end. With the meat, use the connective tissue and dark meats pulled from the bones of your chicken carcass after making stock. They are most healing for the gut.

2 quarts homemade chicken stock (page 10)
2–4 tablespoons animal fat, coconut oil, or ghee
3 carrots, peeled and diced
1 yellow onion, diced (or 1 leek, sliced down the middle, washed, and sliced again into half-moons)
1–2 cups cauliflower, chopped or riced (see page 87)

3 tablespoons fresh parsley, chopped (Stage 2)
1–2 cups leftover roasted or poached chicken meat, chopped or shredded
¼–½ pound liver, chopped finely (optional)
Sea salt
Homemade yogurt (page 27) or cultured cream (page 30), if tolerated (optional)

Combine the stock, fat, and vegetables in a soup pot and bring to a boil. Reduce the heat to a simmer and simmer the soup for at least 15 to 30 minutes or until the vegetables are tender. (At this stage, do not sauté vegetables before adding them. Simmering vegetables is gentler on your digestion, and when combined with good animal fats will start the healing process.) Add the chicken and liver and cook through. Season with sea salt to taste. Serve with homemade yogurt or cultured cream, if tolerated.

Butternut Squash Soup
Serves 6 to 8

I discovered a version of this soup in Jessica Prentice's *Full Moon Feast*. After I made it, I felt like I had become a gourmet chef. Easy, delicious, and a crowd pleaser.

2 quarts chicken stock (page 10)
2 tablespoons animal fat, coconut oil,
  or ghee
3 leeks, sliced in half, and sliced again
  into half-moons (or 2 onions, chopped)

1 butternut squash, peeled, seeded,
  and cut into chunks
1 bouquet garni
Sea salt

Optional Garnishes

Yogurt or cultured cream
Chopped fresh herbs (Stage 2)

Soaked and sprouted pumpkin seeds
  (Full GAPS)

Add the stock and fat to a pot. Add the vegetables and bring to a boil. Reduce the heat to a simmer, add the bouquet garni, and cook, covered, for 30 minutes or until the vegetables are soft and the squash is easily pierced with a fork. Take out the bouquet garni and remove the soup from the heat. Carefully puree the soup with an immersion blender until smooth. Add salt to taste and serve.

Note: *You can substitute filtered water for stock if you don't have enough stock.*

Carrot Ginger Soup
Serves 6 to 8

This warming soup is nice with a dollop of cultured cream and a few sprigs of parsley or cilantro to garnish. (Fresh herbs are allowed in Stage 2.)

2 quarts homemade chicken stock (page 10)
2–4 tablespoons animal fat, coconut oil, or ghee
2 onions, chopped (or 2 leeks, sliced down the middle, then cut into half-moons)

1 pound carrots (about 8–10), peeled and chopped
1 bulb gingerroot, grated (about 3 tablespoons)
Sea salt

Add the stock and fat to a pot. Add the vegetables and ginger and bring to a boil. Reduce the heat to a simmer and cook, covered, for 30 minutes. Puree with an immersion blender until smooth. Add sea salt to taste.

Crock-Pot Beef Soup
Serves 4 to 6

1 quart chicken or beef stock
1 pound stew beef, rump roast, or chuck roast
2–3 tablespoons animal fat, coconut oil, or ghee
1 head kale (stems removed) or Swiss chard
2–4 chopped fresh tomatoes or 1 jar or can (28 ounces) organic whole peeled tomatoes

1 onion, chopped
2 carrots, diced
2 celery stalks, diced (Full GAPS)
2 cloves garlic, pressed
2 sprigs each rosemary and thyme or other fresh herbs (Stage 2)
1 bay leaf
Sea salt

I throw all of the ingredients into my Crock-Pot. It takes all of 5 minutes to chop, stir it around a bit, and press START. Cook slow and low for 4 to 6 hours. If you have a VitaClay (see resources for suppliers), you can do it in 2 hours. You can also use a casserole dish or Dutch oven and place in your oven at 285 to 320°F for 5 to 6 hours. Just add the vegetables 40 to 50 minutes before it's time to eat. Add sea salt to taste. Once you're at Stage 4, you can brown your meat first before adding vegetables.

Maitake Mushroom Immune-Boosting Soup
Serves 6 to 8

This recipe was inspired by my amazing little health food store down the street. It's a healing and nutritious soup with or without the mushrooms. Replace the mushrooms with chicken, fish, pork, or steak if desired.

2 quarts chicken or beef stock
2–3 tablespoons animal fat, coconut oil, or ghee
2–3 maitake mushrooms, chopped
1 tablespoon fresh gingerroot, peeled and minced or finely chopped
5–6 cloves garlic, pressed or chopped

1–2 cups shredded chicken, beef, fish, or pork that has been cooked in stock (optional)
2- to 3-inch piece fresh turmeric, peeled and shredded (optional)
Sea salt
2–3 scallions, chopped (optional)

Bring the stock to a boil. Skim and discard the scum. Place the stock and fat in a large soup pot and bring to a boil. Reduce the heat to a simmer and add the remaining ingredients, except the scallions. Simmer for 30 minutes. Add scallions, cook for another few minutes, and serve.

Onion Soup
Serves 6 to 8

2 quarts chicken or beef stock
3–5 tablespoons animal fat, coconut oil, or ghee
2 leeks, sliced in half, and sliced again into half-moons
2 onions, red and/or white, sliced
2 shallots, sliced

2 cloves garlic, pressed or chopped
1 bouquet garni
Sea salt
1 cup shredded chicken, beef, or meatballs that have been cooked in stock (optional)
Cultured cream (optional)

Bring the stock to a boil. Skim and discard the scum. Add the fat to the pot and bring to a boil. Add the vegetables and turn the heat down to a simmer. Add the bouquet garni, cover, and cook for 30 minutes. Remove the bouquet garni and puree the soup with an immersion blender. Season with sea salt to taste and serve with shredded chicken, beef, or meatballs and a dollop of cultured cream, if desired.

Tomato Soup
Serves 6 to 8

2 quarts chicken stock
2–4 tablespoons animal fat, coconut oil,
  or ghee
8 fresh tomatoes (3–4 cups), chopped, or
  2 jars or cans (28 ounces each) crushed
  tomatoes

2 onions, diced
2 cloves garlic, pressed
1 pound ground pork sausage, crumbled
  (optional)
Sea salt
Handful of fresh basil, shredded (Stage 2)

Bring the stock to a boil. Skim and discard the scum. Add the fat to the pot and bring to a boil. Add the tomatoes, onions, and garlic; turn the heat down to a simmer. Simmer for 20 to 30 minutes, until the onions are soft. Puree with an immersion blender. Add the ground sausage and simmer another 10 minutes. Add salt to taste. Add fresh basil as a garnish in Stage 2.

Variation (Stage 4 or later): Sauté the sausage in the fat until it's nicely browned, about 15 minutes. Remove to a plate. Add the onions to the pan and sauté until translucent. Add the garlic and stir for another minute. Transfer the onions and garlic to the soup pot. Add the stock to the pot, bring to a boil, skim, and discard the scum. Add the tomatoes and simmer for 15 minutes. Puree the soup with an immersion blender—or leave it chunky if you prefer. Add the sausage and stir to incorporate. Let the ingredients simmer together for another 15 minutes. Season with sea salt to taste. Sprinkle with fresh chopped basil to garnish and serve.

Chicken Thighs with Leeks and Mushrooms
Serves 4 to 8

This dish was vital for our family on the GAPS Intro Diet. Our kids scrambled for it, and I was happy to create a meal early on that allowed for a little crispy skin while still cooking the meat in stock. My daughter often has a chicken thigh for breakfast, lunch, and dinner. We triple the amount of chicken that is called for in this recipe for our big family! For the mushrooms, I like to use shiitakes or baby portobellos. Once you reach Stage 2, whisk an egg yolk (or, in Stage 3, a whole egg) into the gelatinous leek-and-mushroom stock for breakfast, or as lunch-on-the-go.

1–2 leeks, sliced in half, and sliced again into half-moons
½ pound mushrooms, stems removed, sliced
4–8 bone-in, skin-on chicken thighs

Sea salt
½–1 quart homemade chicken stock
2 tablespoons animal fat, coconut oil, or ghee

Preheat the oven to 350°F. Scatter the leeks and mushrooms in a big roasting pan. Place the chicken thighs on top, and sprinkle with sea salt. Carefully add the stock to the pan, just high enough to cover the meat with a little skin showing. Add the fat and bake for 30 to 40 minutes. Check once or twice to make sure the leeks and mushrooms are submerged in the stock. Serve with stock or vegetables and salad on the side.

Steak with Mushroom-and-Leek Gravy
Serves 6 to 8

This was a great way for us to have a steak at the beginning of the Intro Diet. See resources for suppliers of quality steaks.

1 quart chicken or beef stock
2 tablespoons animal fat, coconut oil, or ghee
1 pound cremini or baby portobello mushrooms, sliced

2 leeks, sliced in half, and sliced again into half-moons
1–2 pounds sandwich steaks or beef cubes
Sea salt

Place the stock in a pot and bring to a boil, skim, and discard the scum. Add the fat and return to a boil. Add the mushrooms and leeks and reduce the heat to a simmer. Cover and cook for about 15 minutes, until the vegetables are soft. Blend with an immersion blender to make a "gravy." Season the steak with sea salt, turn up the heat under the "gravy," add the meat to the pot, and cook for an additional 2 to 5 minutes. Remove the steaks and place on a plate. Top with mushroom-and-leek gravy. For my kids, I usually cut the steak up and return it to the pot, then serve in bowls.

Ginger Tea with Coconut and Turmeric
Serves 1

When we were going through the GAPS Intro Diet, this was a daily staple, and I often enjoyed it throughout the day. It is a great way to keep blood sugar stabilized as well as a delicious hot drink. You can adjust the amount of ginger and turmeric to your liking.

1 inch gingerroot
½ inch turmeric (optional)
1 cup boiled filtered water

1 teaspoon coconut oil
1 teaspoon raw honey (optional)

Peel and grate the gingerroot and turmeric into a mug; add the hot water. Add the coconut oil and stir. Wait for the tea to cool slightly before adding your raw honey if you wish to preserve the raw enzymes.

Coconut Creams
Serves 12 to 20

½ cup honey

½ cup coconut oil, at room temperature

Whip together the honey and coconut oil with a fork and put into silicone ice cube molds. Place in the freezer for an hour or until solid. Remove from the freezer and pop out as needed, or place them all in a container in the freezer for easy access. You can get creative with the shapes of the molds, which is fun for kids. For added pizzazz, I add freshly grated gingerroot, making it easy to pop into my hot water for an on-the-go ginger tea. These are also a treat eaten as is right out of the freezer. They will satisfy any sweet craving or whiny child.

Note: *If you do not like the taste of coconut oil, you can purchase expeller-pressed oil, which is flavorless. See resources for suppliers.*

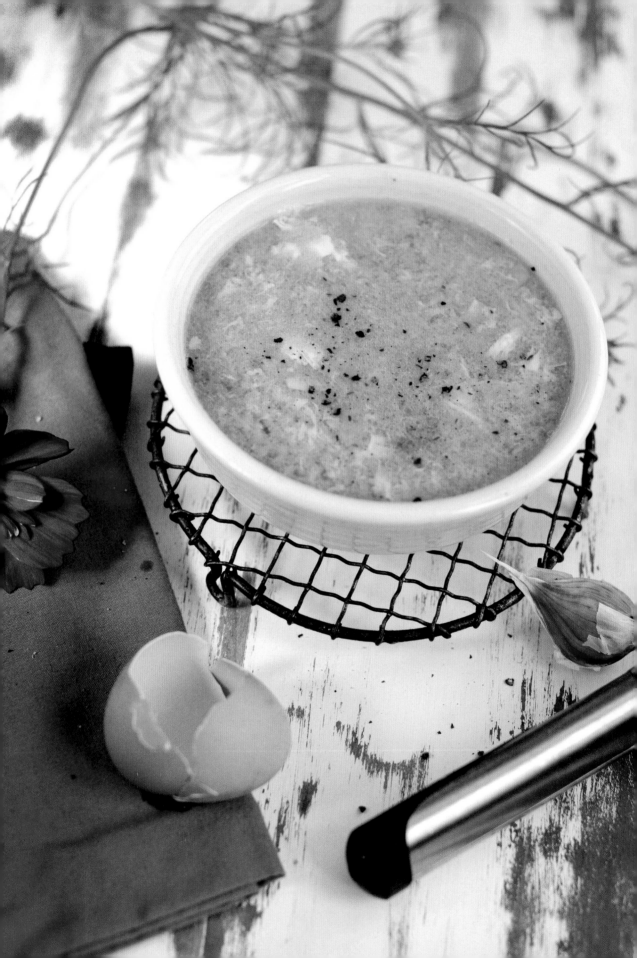

½ cup fresh lime juice

Sea salt

Cultured cream (optional)

Avocado (Stage 3)

Cilantro (Stage 5)

Bring the stock to a boil. Skim and discard the scum. Add the tomato paste and garlic. Add the shredded poached chicken, if you're using it, and simmer for about 30 minutes. Add lime juice and season to taste. Serve with cultured cream, avocado (in Stage 3), or cilantro (Stage 5).

Creamy Cabbage "Casserole" with Chicken Thighs
Serves 4 to 6

I've never really known what to do with cabbage. Since I'd never been a huge fan, it simply wasn't in my repertoire of recipes. Then I discovered Dr. Campbell-McBride's simple "Nice Way to Cook Cabbage" recipe. I have adapted it, and I now am a cooked cabbage lover! This makes great leftovers and gets more and more flavorful each time it is heated up.

1 quart homemade chicken or beef stock

3–5 tablespoons animal fat

½ cabbage, finely sliced

1 large carrot, finely sliced

½ onion, diced

1 tomato, diced

1 tablespoon minced garlic

8 chicken thighs, preferably bone-in with skin on

Sea salt

½ cup cultured cream, kefir, or yogurt (optional)

Preheat the oven to 350°F. Place the stock in an ovenproof pot with the animal fat. Bring to a simmer over medium-high heat. Add the cabbage, carrot, onion, tomato, and garlic. Carefully nestle the chicken thighs into the cabbage, and sprinkle them liberally with sea salt. The skin should just be peeping out of the top of the broth. Cover and cook on medium-low heat on the stovetop for 30 minutes. Remove the cover and put into the oven for an additional 15 minutes, until the chicken skin is golden brown. Serve bowls of soup with accompanying chicken thighs. Add a dollop of cultured cream and enjoy.

Honey Gravlax
Serves 8 to 10

I was initially intimidated to make this, and now I wish I had tried it sooner!

1 2- to 3-pound plank wild salmon
1 bunch fresh dill
1 bunch fresh cilantro
¼ cup chopped chives

¾ cups coarse sea salt
¼ cup raw honey
Zest of 2 lemons
1 tablespoon ground peppercorns

Wash the salmon and pat it dry. Place it on a cutting board and cut into two pieces. In one mixing bowl combine the fresh herbs, and in another combine the salt, honey, lemon zest, and ground pepper.

On a clean plate, place a third of the herb mix. Place the salmon skin side down on top of the herbs, and coat the top with half the honey-and-salt mixture. Add another layer of fresh herbs followed by the second piece of salmon skin side up. Add the remainder of the salt mixture followed by the remainder of the herb mixture. Cover in plastic wrap. Top with a small cutting board or plate with a weighted pot on top to weigh down the fish. Let chill in the fridge for 16 to 24 hours.

Gently wash or rub off the salt and herbs and pat the salmon dry. Skin it, slice thinly on the diagonal, and serve. This is delicious with fresh dill, capers, chopped pickles, and diced red onion (Stage 5). This will make a salmon lover out of anyone, even kids!

Boiled Meatballs and Burgers
Serves 4 to 6

This is still not quite the burger from the past, but you are getting close.

1 quart stock or soup of any kind
1 pound ground meat: beef, lamb, pork, chicken, or turkey, including ground organs, if desired

2 egg yolks
1 clove garlic, pressed (optional)
1 teaspoon sea salt

Pour the stock (or soup) into a large skillet. Cover and bring to a simmer over medium-low heat. Meanwhile, gently mix the remaining ingredients together in a bowl. Roll into balls or form into patties and gently place them into the skillet with the broth. Simmer, covered, until cooked through or to your liking, about 5 to 15 minutes. Eat as is, with the soup, or save the soup or stock for future sipping!

Cabbage and Sausage Stew
Serves 8 to 10

I have always loved this recipe, and I was dying to re-create it for GAPS. This originates from Jessica Prentice's *Full Moon Feast*, and it is delicious!

½–1 cup stock
2 tablespoons lard or other animal fat
2 leeks (or onions), sliced in half, and sliced again into half-moons
1 small head cabbage or ½ large head, shredded
1 bunch greens such as spinach, chard, kale, collards, mustard, turnip, or radish, sliced into ribbons

1–2 small rutabagas or turnips, diced
Sea salt
1–2 pounds whole fresh sausages in casings
½ cup sauerkraut
Cultured cream (optional)

Put the stock in your pot and add the animal fat. Add the leeks, shredded cabbage, greens, rutabagas, and a good pinch of sea salt. Bring to a simmer, cover, and cook over medium-low heat until the rutabagas are easily pierced with a fork, about 15 minutes. Slip the sausages from their casings into the pot and break up with a wooden spoon. Continue cooking for 15 minutes to allow the sausage to cook through. Add more stock as needed. Add plenty of sea salt to taste. Serve in individual bowls. As the soup cools, stir in the sauerkraut and a generous amount of cultured cream.

Variation (Stage 4): Heat the animal fat in a pot and sauté the leeks for 10 minutes. Add the shredded cabbage and a pinch of salt. Sauté until the cabbage starts to wilt. Add the greens, and stir to incorporate. Add the rutabagas and another pinch of salt, followed by a splash of stock. Cover the pot, reduce the heat to a simmer, and steam the rutabagas until they are easily pierced with a fork. Add more stock as needed if it gets too dry. Slip the sausages from their casings into the pot and break up with a wooden spoon. Continue cooking for 15 minutes to allow the sausage to cook through. Add plenty of salt to taste. Serve in individual bowls. As the soup cools, stir in the sauerkraut and a generous amount of cultured cream.

Basic Beef Stew
Serves 8 to 10

Stews are a welcome addition in Stage 2. It's so nice to finally be able to have something a little more substantial than soup alone. If you're purchasing cow parts in bulk, this is a great way to use the tougher cuts of meat such as roasts and chuck. At the market, you'll often find them with the label STEWING BEEF. You can substitute chicken breast for the stew meat.

2–3 pounds cubed stew meat or a round roast	5 cups chopped vegetables, such as carrots and onions
Sea salt	Homemade chicken or beef stock, just to cover

Take the meat out of the fridge and let it come to room temperature; season generously with sea salt. Place the meat and vegetables in a pot. Add stock to almost cover everything. (If you're short on stock, you can supplement with filtered water.) Bring to a boil, then reduce the heat to a simmer. Cover and cook for about 45 minutes, or until all the vegetables are soft. If you're using a roast, carefully remove it from the pot to a cutting board. First slice with a chef's knife, then shred it with two forks. Return the meat to the stew, and add sea salt to taste. For a variation try topping this with Mashed Cauliflower (recipe follows).

Note: *You can also cook the round roast in a slow cooker on low for 6 to 8 hours or even roast it in the oven at a low temperature (250°F, covered, for 2 to 3 hours) with the vegetables and stock. The slow cooker is my preferred method of cooking since the meat just falls apart when finished. If you have 10 minutes in the morning to prep, dinner simply involves adding a few ferments, some cultured cream, and some chopped avocado on top!*

Variation (Stage 4): Take your meat out of the fridge 1 hour before cooking, allow it to come to room temperature, and season generously with sea salt. And fresh black pepper. Melt ¼ cup animal fat (I recommend tallow) over medium-high heat in a Dutch oven on the stovetop and brown the meat. After the meat is browned, remove it to a plate, then put your vegetables of choice into the Dutch oven.

Stir the vegetables to coat with the meat's juices, adding 2 tablespoons fresh thyme or 2 teaspoons dried thyme (Stage 5), 2 to 3 crushed garlic cloves, 2 to 3 bay leaves, and a pinch of sea salt. Cook for about 5 minutes, then return the meat to the Dutch oven. Add stock to almost cover everything. (If you're short on stock, you can supplement with filtered water.) Bring to a boil, then reduce the heat to a simmer. Cover and cook for about 45 minutes, or until all the vegetables are soft. Follow instructions above.

Mashed Cauliflower
Serves 6 to 8

After getting the hang of Basic Stew, you can create casseroles by transferring the stew to an ovenproof dish, adding Mashed Cauliflower on top, and cooking in the oven at 350°F for about 30 minutes. This is similar to a shepherd's pie.

1 head cauliflower

3–4 cups filtered water or stock

3–4 tablespoons ghee, coconut oil, lard, or tallow

Sea salt

1–2 tablespoons cultured cream and/or ghee

Break up the cauliflower into little florets. Steam it or bring it to a boil in the filtered water or stock, then reduce the heat to a simmer for 10 to 15 minutes. Strain and place back into the hot pot. Add the fat of your choice and blend with a handheld blender, or transfer to a food processor and blend until soft and smooth. Add cultured cream and/or ghee and salt to taste.

Ground Beef Stew
Serves 8 to 10

This is a delicious variation on traditional beef stew. It's great with a fried egg on top. For the ground beef, I use 1 pound with organs, 1 pound without. This stew can also be made with ground chicken, turkey, pork, or lamb. And it's excellent as a casserole with Mashed Cauliflower (above) on top.

1–2 quarts beef stock
3 onions, diced
2 celery stalks, diced
2 carrots, diced
2–3 tablespoons lard, beef tallow, or
    other fat

2 pounds ground beef
2 sprigs fresh rosemary, chopped
2 sprigs fresh thyme
4–5 fresh sage leaves, chopped
1 bay leaf
1–2 teaspoons sea salt

Add the stock, vegetables, and animal fat to your pot. Bring to a boil, and turn the heat down to a simmer. Add the meat, breaking it apart with a wooden spoon. Add the herbs and cover. Simmer on low for 45 minutes. Add sea salt to taste, and serve it up in bowls.

Variation (Stage 4): Generously season the beef with sea salt. In a Dutch oven or stew pot, brown the beef in the fat. Remove the meat to a bowl. In the same pot, sauté the onions, celery, and carrots with a pinch of sea salt, adding more fat if needed. Add the herbs, and sauté for 20 to 25 minutes on medium-low, allowing the flavors to infuse the vegetables and caramelize slightly. Return the ground beef and its juices to the pot, and continue cooking for 5 more minutes, stirring to incorporate. Add the beef stock and turn the heat down. Simmer, covered, for 45 minutes. Serve it up in bowls.

Salted Caramels

These were another of my family's favorites while we were on the Intro Diet. Use equal parts honey and ghee, adding a pinch of sea salt. Place in silicone ice cube trays or chocolate molds. For additional ideas, see Coconut Creams (page 51). Enjoy right out of the freezer or in a cup of tea!

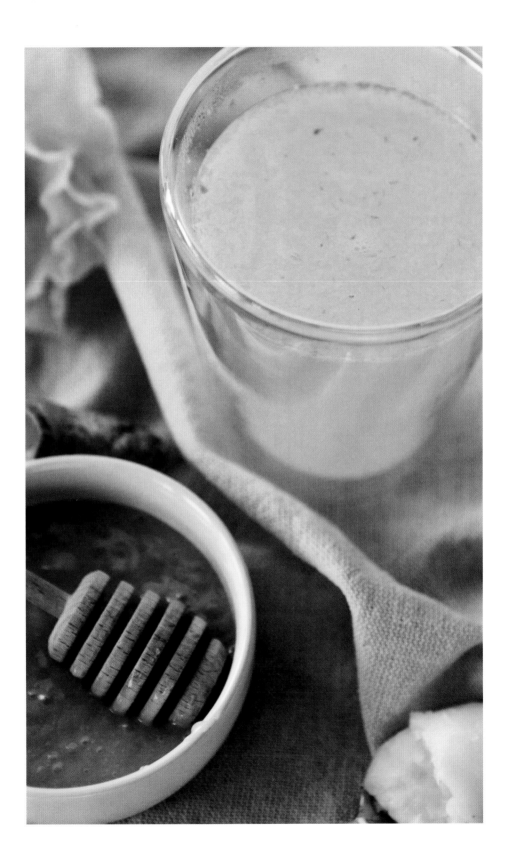

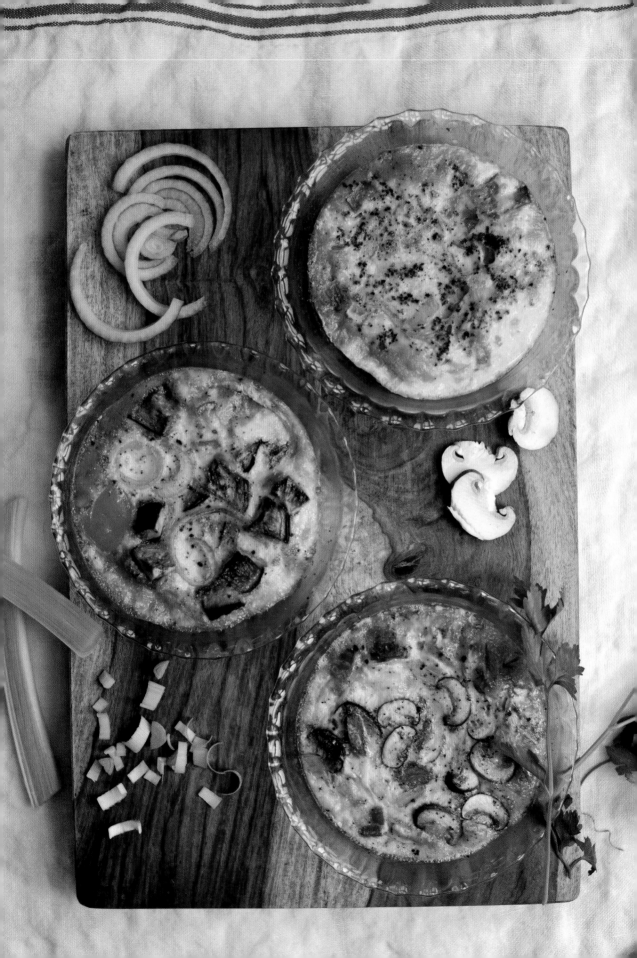

S tage 3 was a big jump for us. Avocado. Read: *guacamole*! We had died and gone to heaven! Avocado was such a welcome addition, and to this day it accompanies nearly every meal we have: breakfast, lunch, and dinner. Mash with a pinch of salt and a squeeze of fresh lime juice, and the kids will devour it. And squash pancakes with a little raw honey on top? Sure, they don't really resemble those fluffy pancakes of the past, but they are delicious and satisfying.

Two eggs, 2 to 3 tablespoons of ginger carrots, two or three squash pancakes, half an avocado (mashed with a pinch of sea salt), plus a bowl of broth with a pinch of salt and a spoonful of lard became our staple breakfast. In addition, eggs all different ways—like omelets overflowing with chicken, avocado, diced tomatoes, and fermented salsa and hot sauce. We had made it through the hardest part. Life was returning to normal or, as my husband likes to say, "our normal." Sure, the little honey treats continued in between meals, as well as our tea with coconut oil, and mainly soups for lunch and dinner. But we were progressing, and we were ecstatic.

Even our brave daughter savored her relatively minimalist daily chicken thigh with crispy skin, onions cooked in loads of fat, and side of homemade guacamole. Her seizures were decreasing every day. The re-introduction of ghee caused them to increase again, so it was promptly removed. In Stage 3, you can anticipate lots of "testing the waters."

On that note, be super mindful at this point. You have achieved a beautifully neutral, non-allergenic state. So watch for any changes as you add things into your diet. A daily diary is a good idea, although I personally didn't stick with this, since I was putting most of my energy into keeping everything and everyone in the house moving—including seven digestive tracts! Indeed, at the beginning of GAPS, things can get quite sluggish—or the opposite may occur. This is normal as your body adjusts, but take measures to keep things moving right along. Home enema kits, dolomite powder, and colonics were among the remedies we entertained, but digestion soon kicked in, at which point I was ready to yodel from the rooftops! In the event of bowels all revved up or stalled out: If you've introduced dairy, then cultured cream and fermented vegetable juices are best for constipation. Likewise, homemade yogurt and whey are best for diarrhea.

As incongruous as it seems to talk about poop in a cookbook, it is vitally important. And as Nick says, once again, "Poop is what makes the world go around." There is nothing worse than an out-of-balance digestive system; we have all been there. I once heard at a Weston A. Price conference that if you have to think about it, then something ain't right, as I sat there downing my fourth cup of tea, hoping to get things moving. I knew "in my gut" that I fit into that category. So keep doing what you are doing, and this, too, shall pass.

Foods Allowed During Stage 3

Continue with previous stage foods. Avocado is a wonderful addition in Stage 3. Start slowly and add it to every meal, mashed or diced. Start to incorporate sautéed onion with lots of animal fat, since it's great for the digestion and the immune system. Continue with fermented vegetables and juices with every meal. At this stage you can go ahead and eat the fermented vegetables along with the juice. Fermented ginger carrots, salsa, and pickles were the favorites in our house.

Introduce therapeutic probiotics on an empty stomach, preferably twenty minutes before eating.

In Stage 3, you can add:
- **Ripe avocado:** Add to soups, starting with 1 to 3 teaspoons and gradually increasing daily
- **Pancakes** made with squash, nut butter (optional), eggs, and a small amount of honey: Start with one per day to start and slowly increase from there
- **Almond butter**
- **Eggs:** soft-boiled, gently fried, or scrambled eggs cooked in plenty of animal fat, ghee, or coconut oil
- **Fully cooked vegetables:** cabbage, celeriac, asparagus
- Sautéed **onion** in lots of animal fat
- GAPS-legal, therapeutic **probiotics** (see resources)
- **Fermented vegetables:** Start with a small amount and increase to 1 to 4 teaspoons per meal

Eggs

Eggs, eggs, and more eggs. I never imagined that we'd be going through ten dozen a week! On the GAPS Intro Diet, putting a yolk or two into every bowl of soup really pumped up our consumption. We still have eggs daily since they are super nutritious and make for an economical meal—breakfast, lunch, or dinner—with leftover vegetables or salad. I still drop eggs in my soups, use yolks to make mayo every week, and add them to my kids' smoothies and juice. Find the very best eggs available. Organic, soy-free, and pastured are the best. If there's a farm down the road that meets these parameters, that's where you should buy them!

Mexican Omelet
Serves 1

On the Intro Diet, I made lots of omelets, especially for my two older boys. They were particularly fond of Mexican omelets. Of course, with eggs, the possibilities for combining great ingredients are endless, but since this one is apparently "awesome!" here is Campbell's and Cooper's favorite Mexican Omelet recipe.

2–4 tablespoons animal fat, ghee, or
    coconut oil
2–3 eggs
Sea salt
¼ cup prepared ground beef (with organs
    is a bonus) or chicken simmered in broth
    with ½ chopped onion, salt, and pepper

¼ cup chopped tomatoes (Stage 5)
2 tablespoons mashed avocado
2 tablespoons Lacto-Fermented
    Cilantro Salsa (page 234)
2 tablespoons chopped cilantro
Cultured cream (optional)

Melt the fat in a hot frying pan. Whisk together the eggs and pour into the frying pan. Distribute the eggs by moving your pan around. Let it firm up a bit, sprinkle with salt, and cook almost through and until it's golden on the bottom. Using a rubber spatula, work around the edges and slide onto a plate. Don't worry if it's not cooked all the way; it will cook when you fold it in half. Fill one half with the ground meat, chopped tomatoes, mashed avocado, Fermented Salsa, and cilantro. Fold the omelet in half. Garnish with a little cultured cream on top, if appropriate.

    As we moved through the stages and could add spices, I would throw in a bit of my Taco Seasoning (page 128) while cooking the meat (Stage 5). On the Full GAPS Diet, we added raw shredded cheese as well. (See the Frittata section in Stage 4 for more ideas, page 77.)

Soft-Boiled Eggs

I remember eating soft-boiled eggs as a kid, with hot buttered toast, a pinch of salt, and some fresh cracked pepper. Yum! Well, bread is no longer in the picture, but the butter and salt are still plenty delicious. On Full GAPS my boys enjoy three soft-boiled eggs, 1 tablespoon raw butter, 1 piece of Coconut Butter Bread (page 118), a slice of avocado, a slice or two of bacon—and salt and pepper, of course.

Fill a saucepan three-quarters of the way with water and bring it to a boil. Throw in a pinch of salt to help prevent the shells from cracking. Using a large spoon or ladle, lower eggs slowly into the boiling water. Remove the pan from the heat, cover, and allow the eggs to cook according to the following timetable:

7 minutes	slightly firm
12 minutes	hard-boiled

When your eggs are ready, run cold water directly into the pan until the shells are cool enough to touch. Crack the eggs in half with a knife and scoop into a bowl with butter and salt.

For hard-boiled eggs, submerge them in a bowl of cold water for 5 minutes to stop the cooking, drain, and place in the fridge.

Fried Eggs

Fried eggs are probably the most popular in our house. They're quick, easy, and perfect with a side of tomato and avocado and a glass of kefir before school.

Season the pan liberally with fat, crack a few eggs into the pan, and cook on medium-low for a few minutes. Keep the heat low so as not to be too hard on their delicate proteins. Sunny-side up is great, as the yolk doesn't get cooked too much. Over easy is, too; just flip for a few seconds, flip back over, and serve.

If my kids are ever hungry before bed, which can happen after an evening game of Capture the Flag, I quickly fry up a few eggs for a snack. Couldn't be easier!

Scrambled Eggs

Whisk eggs in a bowl. Melt fat in your frying pan, over low heat, and pour in the eggs. Stir gently and scrape the sides with a wooden spoon. When the eggs are still a bit runny, remove from the pan and sprinkle with salt. They will continue to cook a bit, so be sure to take them out on the earlier side.

Poached Eggs

Poached eggs can be tricky, but they are delicious. My mom frequently made eggs Benedict for dinner. That was a favorite, for sure. In her honor, I've often re-created that meal with toasted Coconut Butter Bread (Full GAPS, page 118), bacon (Full GAPS), a poached egg, avocado, and hollandaise sauce (page 111) . . . even she approves! For breakfast Nick often poaches two eggs in stock and adds sausage into the broth (or cooks it on the side before adding), along with a little fermented hot sauce (page 241).

To poach an egg, place a good-sized skillet on the stove filled with water and add a pinch of salt. Bring to a simmer. Crack an egg into a cup or bowl, and slowly pour it into the hot water. It will look a little feathery, but don't worry. Cook your eggs for 2 to 4 minutes depending on the firmness you desire. Remove from the pan with a slotted spoon and smother in ghee. On Full GAPS, place the eggs on Coconut Butter Bread smothered in ghee or bacon grease. Eat as is or add any additions you wish. Salmon, hollandaise sauce, and a little fresh dill is killer; or try avocado, bacon, and hollandaise. Always remember a nice pinch of sea salt and fresh cracked pepper (Stage 5)!

Squash Pancakes
Makes 6 to 8 small pancakes

My kids love these with a little butter or ghee and a tiny bit of honey on top. They are fairly sweet without the honey, so only add if your kids are demanding it!

1 cup cooked squash, pureed
   (recipe follows)
3 pastured eggs
1 teaspoon cinnamon (Stage 5)

1 teaspoon vanilla extract (homemade
   only; see recipe, page 96)
Pinch of sea salt
2 tablespoons animal fat, coconut oil, or
   ghee (for cooking)

Blend the first five ingredients in a bowl. Pour about ¼ cup of batter for each pancake into a pan with lots of melted fat. Let cook for a minute or two on the first side, then flip. It takes a little bit to get the hang of it since they are small, but just don't flip too soon or they will fall apart.

Squash Puree

To make your squash puree, cut any winter squash (butternut, acorn, pumpkin) half lengthwise and scoop out the seeds. Place facedown on a jelly-roll with a little water to cover the bottom of the pan. Roast in a 350°F oven for 45 minutes or until your fork sinks right through the flesh. Remove from the oven and let cool. Scoop out the flesh, and place in your food processor. Process until smooth. When the puree is cool, store in 2-cup servings in ziplock bags stacked in the freezer.

Celery Root Soup
Serves 6 to 8

I had a few celery roots in my CSA box a few months back, and I decided to re-create the celery root soup I had just happened to have twice in the last week at a great local restaurant, 80 Thoreau, adapted to make it GAPS-legal. To keep it simple in the beginning, just add the mushrooms to your soup to cook after you've pureed the other ingredients. If you suffer from candida, you may want to hold off on the mushrooms until you clear that up.

2 quarts chicken stock	2 celery roots, peeled and cubed
2–3 tablespoons animal fat, coconut oil, or ghee	2 leeks, washed and sliced
	1 fennel bulb, chopped
2 onions, chopped	Sea salt

Bring the stock to a boil in a big soup pot, skim, and discard the scum. Add the fat and bring to a simmer. Add all the vegetables and continue to simmer, covered, until soft (about 20 minutes). Puree the soup with an immersion blender, and add salt to taste.

Garnish with Sautéed Garlicky Mushrooms (page 75) and a drizzle of olive oil, once you're on Stage 4.

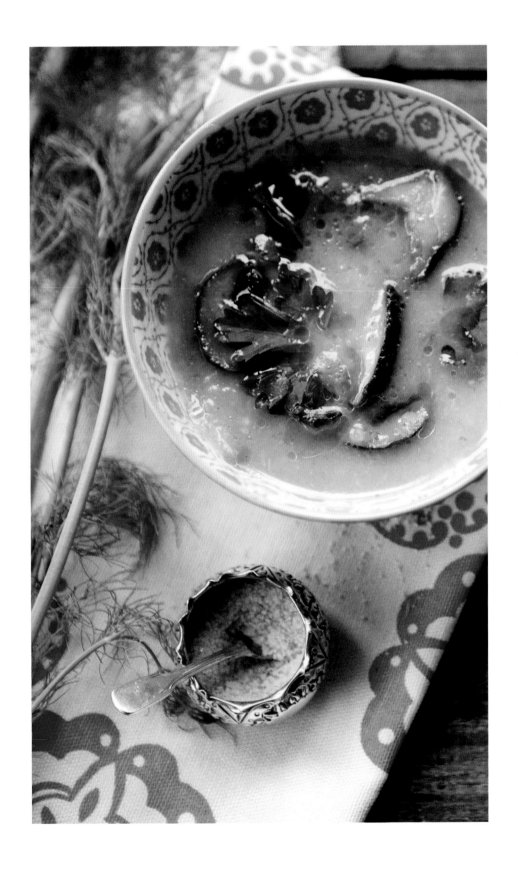

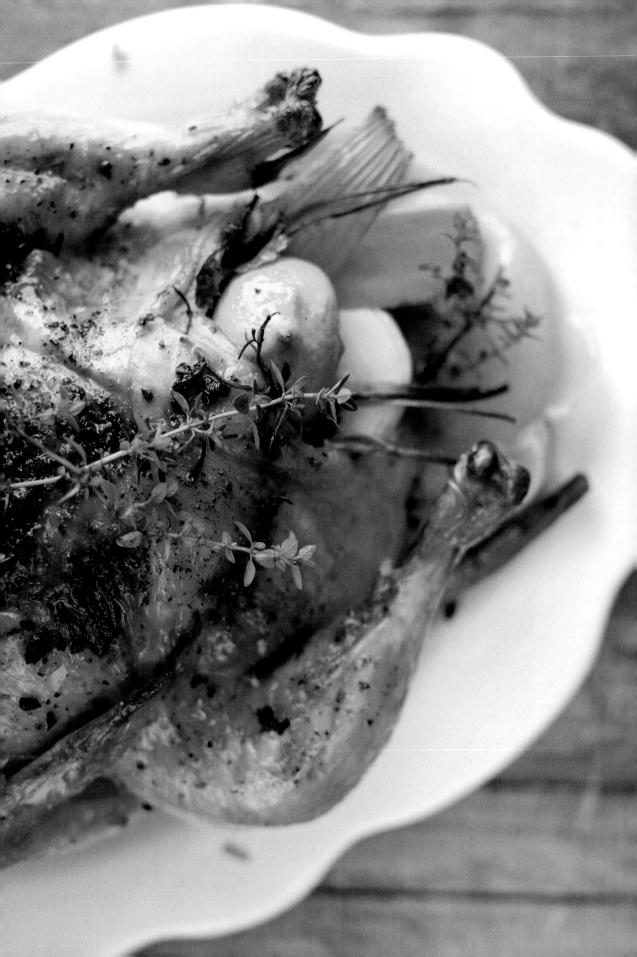

N ick is just full of wisdom. As he said to another father who was seriously doubting the GAPS protocol after painfully watching his kids' lethargy and sickness throughout the first week: "Just make it to the burger, dude. Just make it to the burger!" For most meat-loving men, the arrival of a burger (not boiled, that is) is totally "clutch"—which, as defined by Urban Dictionary, means, "Exactly what you need, exactly when you need it." A burger with garlic aioli, caramelized onions, and garlicky mushrooms could be anyone's perfect meal, whether they're on GAPS or not. Eat one of those, and you'll see that all your anxiety and nervousness about being on this diet, all your doubts and fears about making it through, were unnecessary. Yes, there is definitely a period of adjustment and inconvenience, but hang tight, stay busy, and keep at it. Things are shifting, and you are laying the groundwork for a future of good health.

As always, keep in mind that the point at which anyone moves from one stage to the next depends on the individual. Don't be discouraged if you need a little extra time in a certain stage. You will know that you do if any unusual symptoms flare with the introduction of new foods: hives, unusual behavior, fatigue, bloating, rashes, the runs, what have you. Just take a step back and simplify your diet again; I know it's hard, but don't rush it, and remember that healing is happening. Our GAPS practitioner texted me at the six-month mark: "Patience!" I wrote back, "Yes, I now see that this is going to be a two-year commitment for us. What a big lesson in patience and love." She replied: "For sure! And you can do it . . . We moms can do anything for our babies!" Again, the Urban Dictionary hooked me up with its spot-on description of *patience*: a requirement for raising children; a relationship; learning; life; achieving anything; conversation. And I would have to add my own: making it to the burger in Stage 4!

Another huge component of Stage 4 is adding in juicing. Juicing is a time-honored tradition for removing toxins from the body, and it's a surefire way to pack a lot of nutrition into one punch! Most often GAPS patients have a toxic overload since their own detoxification systems are not up to speed. Our natural detoxification systems require many of the nutrients in which GAPS patients are deficient. Juicing at this stage can help our bodies start to remove the toxic overload that hinders healing.

The addition of juicing was certainly a curveball for our family since we did not have a juicer and juicing for seven people translates to a lot of money spent on organic vegetables. We tried the Vitamix/straining thing for about a month—until Mother's Day, when I got a juicer on sale at Macy's. I guess you could say that the traditional breakfast-in-bed and day spent doting on Mom fell by the wayside when I found myself alone at the mall, purchasing an appliance in order to spend yet more time in the kitchen! Oh, the irony.

It was worth it, though. Juicing is a super-effective way to speed your body's detoxification. But don't feel like you won't heal if you miss a day or two (or five) of juicing. Yes, it is a fabulous part of the program, but it does require effort and can be expensive. If you don't have enough time or resources to do it regularly, just do it when you can. My GAPS practitioner assured me that stressing about it was worse than not juicing. I went strong for the first three months, and then summer arrived and we began eating more fresh vegetables. I eased up on the juicing for a bit, and then ratcheted things back up come fall.

Foods Allowed During Stage 4

Continue with previous stage foods. At this point you may start to simmer your stocks for longer, add roasted and baked meats, olive oil, and nut flour breads. Be sure to add plenty of ghee to each slice of bread.

In Stage 4, you can add:

- **Roasted and baked meats, including fish** (not barbecued or fried): Add gradually
- **Cold-pressed olive oil:** Start with a few drops and increase to 1 to 2 tablespoons per meal
- **Fresh-pressed juices:** Start with 1 teaspoon per day of fresh carrot juice on an empty stomach, then add celery, lettuce, and mint
- **Walnut and almond flour**
- **Breads made with nut and seed flours**

Burgers with Garlic Aioli and Caramelized Onions
Serves 8

Delicious! What a milestone!

4 tablespoons ghee, coconut oil, or
  lard, divided
2–3 onions, sliced
Sea salt

Honey, optional
2 pounds ground beef (great place to add
  in ground organs)
Garlic Aioli (page 108)

To make the caramelized onions, add 2 tablespoons of the fat to a pan. Add the sliced onions with a few pinches of sea salt. Cook over medium-low for 30 minutes until caramelized. A touch of honey stirred in at the end adds a nice sweetness to the onions if you'd like. Remove the onions from the pan to a serving dish.

Form your beef into patties, being careful not to work them too much. Generously add sea salt to both sides. Add the remaining 2 tablespoons of fat to your pan, and cook the burgers; for a medium-rare burger, this takes about 4 minutes per side over medium heat. Top with Garlic Aioli and Sautéed Garlicky Mushrooms (below), and serve alongside some fermented vegetables.

Sautéed Garlicky Mushrooms
Serves 4 to 6

These are just amazing, with anything from soup to eggs to burgers to tenderloin. If you like mushrooms, these are quick, easy, and delicious (my mantra). I usually combine baby portobellos and shiitakes, but you can do whatever is most economical given the season and what's available. You can even buy dried mushrooms; just reconstitute them in water for half an hour before using. Remember that mushrooms shrink a lot when cooked, so buy more than you think you'll need, especially if you have mushroom lovers in the house.

1–2 pounds mushrooms
2 tablespoons animal fat, coconut oil, or ghee (butter is delicious, too, when tolerated)

Sea salt
2 garlic cloves, pressed or chopped finely
Handful of chopped parsley

Clean off the mushrooms with a dish towel to remove any dirt. Remove the stems and slice. Add the fat to a pan, and throw in the mushrooms with a pinch of salt. Sauté for about 10 minutes, add the garlic, and continue to cook on low for another 5 to 10 minutes. Add salt to taste, sprinkle with fresh parsley, and serve!

Roasted Chicken
Serves 6 to 8

1 3- to 5-pound pasture-raised chicken
3 onions
3 carrots, cut in half
Generous pinch of sea salt
1 lemon

1 celery stalk, cut in half
2–3 cloves garlic, whole
Fresh herbs like parsley, thyme, and
    rosemary (whatever you have on hand)
¼ cup lard, coconut oil, or ghee

Rinse the chicken and pat it dry. Slice 2 of the onions, chop 2 of the carrots, and spread these out over the bottom of a roasting pan or a baking dish. Stuff the chicken with a big pinch of salt, half the lemon, half of the remaining onion, the remaining carrot, the celery, the garlic, and the fresh herbs (I love fresh thyme), followed by the other half onion and lemon (if you can fit them). Then place the chicken in the pan atop your onions and carrots.

Rub the fat over the chicken and under the skin; smear a few dollops on top, too. Sprinkle generously with unrefined sea salt as well as more of any herbs you have around.

Roast at 375°F for 1½ to 3 hours (depending on the chicken's size). Halfway through, stir the vegetables around the chicken. Using a meat thermometer, check the temperature in the thickest part of the chicken breast. When it reads 160°F, or the juices run clear when the breast is pierced with a fork, remove the pan from the oven. Allow the roasted chicken to rest for about 10 minutes before carving. Serve alongside the caramelized onions and carrots from the bottom of the pan, pouring the pan juices over everything.

Giblet Gravy for Roasted Chicken
Serves 6 to 8

My grandmother always made giblet gravy, although none of us ever thought about the fact that we were eating organ meats. It was so tasty we didn't care!

Always remove the bag of giblets from inside your chicken's cavity before roasting. You can start cooking them on the stovetop while your bird is in the oven. A great leftover option is to toast a piece of Coconut Butter Bread (page 118), butter it generously, then top with chicken and a drizzle of gravy.

Giblets and pan juices from 1 roasted
    chicken

1–2 tablespoons gelatin (optional)
Sea salt

Remove the giblets from the chicken, rinse, and place in a small pot of filtered water. Bring to a boil and skim the top. Reduce the heat to a simmer and leave for 10 to 15 minutes. Once the giblets are cooked through, you can take them out and let them cool.

In the meantime, roast your chicken. You will have wonderful drippings on the bottom of the pan. Remove the roasted chicken to a serving platter. Then pop your pan right on the stovetop, and bring the chicken juices to a boil.

On a cutting board, chop and mash up your giblets, removing any tough membranes. Add them to the pan juices and continue to mash with a fork or the back of a wooden spoon. Let the paste brown a bit in the pan, then slowly add the giblets' cooking water to the pan, about ¼ cup at a time, until the gravy reaches your desired consistency (you can substitute chicken stock). Turn down the heat and stir out all of the lumps with the back of a wooden spoon or whisk.

If you would like to thicken the gravy a bit, add the gelatin 1 tablespoon at a time (this will not be a thick gravy like you are used to). Upon finishing the gravy, you can use an immersion blender to get the texture nice and smooth if you wish. Add sea salt to taste!

Serve over chicken.

Frittata
Serves 4 to 6

Frittatas are a wonderful way to feed a crowd and our go-to for using up leftover vegetables for breakfast, lunch, or dinner. I often make these when we have a breakfast celebration at my kids' school. Again, the potential flavor combinations are endless; try incorporating any of the meats and/or vegetable combinations listed below.

2–4 tablespoons lard, coconut oil, or ghee

1 cup cooked meats and/or vegetables of choice

6–8 pastured eggs

2 pinches of sea salt

Raw cheese (optional, Full GAPS)

Fresh herbs (optional)

Turn on the broiler or preheat the oven to 350°F. Over medium heat, melt half the fat of your choice in an ovenproof frying pan (I love my cast-iron pan), making sure to coat the bottom and sides. Toss in whatever vegetables you're using and sauté for 5 minutes. Remove to a plate.

Add the second half of the fat to the pan. Whisk the eggs, season with sea salt, and pour into the pan. Scatter the vegetables and meat on top. Reduce the heat to medium-low. Using a wooden spoon, gently lift the sides of the frittata to let uncooked egg run underneath until set, approximately 5 minutes. Place the frittata in the oven until it's slightly golden and set, 2 to 3 minutes under the broiler or 5 to 10 minutes in a 350°F oven. Sprinkle with fresh herbs if you like; on Full GAPS, grate raw cheese (Parmesan is delicious) on top as well.

Variations: Get creative with frittatas! Here are a few ideas to get you started:
- Sausage, mushroom, and leek.
- Leftover roasted vegetables with sausage (our favorite). I always roast extra vegetables at night and make a frittata the next morning for breakfast or lunch.
- Salmon, spinach. and red onion. This is a great way to use up leftover fish.
- Roasted peppers, red onion, and eggplant.
- Sea salt and fresh cracked pepper (Stage 5) are always a must.

Pan-Seared Scallops
Serves 4 to 6

4 tablespoons ghee or fat of choice, divided
20–24 sea scallops, rinsed and patted dry, then seasoned with sea salt
2 cloves garlic, pressed

Handful of fresh parsley, chopped
Juice from ½ lemon
½ cup dry white wine (Full GAPS)
½ pound sugar-free bacon, cooked and chopped (optional, Full GAPS)

In a large skillet over medium-high heat, add 2 tablespoons of the fat. When the pan is hot but not smoking, add as many scallops as you can, without crowding the pan, along with the garlic; cook for 1½ to 2 minutes per side. Remove from the pan, and cook the remaining scallops, adding more fat as needed. Sprinkle with chopped parsley and a squeeze of lemon juice, and serve. On Full GAPS, deglaze the pan with a splash of white wine upon flipping the scallops. Top with chopped bacon and fresh parsley.

Stuffed Peppers
Serves 6

This is a great way to use up leftovers and peppers from your garden or a vegetable CSA.

6 peppers (any color), summer squash,
   or zucchini
2 tablespoons animal fat
2 cups riced cauliflower (page 87)
1 pound ground sausage, or leftover
   chicken or beef
1 onion, diced
2 cloves garlic, pressed

1 pound mushrooms, sliced (optional)
2 handfuls spinach
A few teaspoons of fresh herbs: thyme,
   rosemary, and oregano
1 teaspoon sea salt
¼ cup toasted pine nuts (Full GAPS)
Raw Parmesan (Full GAPS)

Preheat the oven to 350°F. Carefully remove the stems from the peppers; slice in half lengthwise to make boats, or simply carve out a hole in the top. (If you're using summer squash or zucchini, slice in half and scrape out the seeds to make a "hollow boat.") Remove the seeds and white membrane from inside the peppers. In a heavy skillet, over medium-low heat, melt a few tablespoons fat and add the riced cauliflower and meat. Add the onion, garlic, mushrooms, spinach, and fresh herbs, and season with sea salt. Sauté for 10 to 15 minutes until soft and flavors are incorporated. Set the peppers in a well-greased baking dish; fill each with stuffing. Bake for 30 to 45 minutes.

    In the meantime, if you're on Full GAPS, toast the pine nuts in a small pan over medium heat for a few minutes until lightly golden (watch closely and shake the pan often; they burn easily). When you remove the baked peppers from the oven, top with toasted pine nuts and freshly grated raw Parmesan.

Almond Flour Bread or Muffins
Makes 1 loaf or 12 muffins

This recipe is great for a treat, especially during the GAPS Intro, but I wouldn't make it an everyday staple. The polyunsaturated oils in almonds are sensitive to heat, which causes them to break down when baked; therefore, they are not optimally nutritious. Enjoy for special occasions.

2 ½ cups ground crispy almonds
(or nut of choice)
2 cups butternut squash puree (page 70)
or applesauce (optional)
4 pastured eggs

¼ cup coconut oil, lard, or ghee, slightly
melted, with an additional 1 tablespoon
for greasing pan or tin
1 teaspoon sea salt

Preheat the oven to 300°F. Grease a loaf pan or muffin tin very well, or set liners into the tin. Grind almonds in a food processor to a fine flour. Be careful not to process too long, or you will end up with almond butter! Transfer the nut flour to a bowl, and add the remaining ingredients. Mix with a hand mixer until the batter is well incorporated, and pour into your pan or tin. Place in the oven and bake for 50 minutes, or until a toothpick when inserted comes out clean. (Muffins cook for 20 minutes or until a toothpick comes out clean.)

Note: *You can also use this basic bread recipe as a pizza crust. Pour the batter onto a well-greased jelly-roll pan in 4- to 5-inch circles, spreading each one out with the back of a spoon. Bake for 30 minutes. Allow to cool before adding sauce and toppings, then return to the oven for 10 to 20 minutes.*

Juices

In Stage 4 start with carrot juice only, and dilute it with warm filtered water or fresh yogurt or whey. Then add celery, lettuce, and mint. Start by "chewing the juice" and work up to 1 cup per day. (Chewing your juice—all foods, for that matter—starts digestion in your mouth, making the process easier.) Try to drink juice on an empty stomach 20 to 25 minutes before eating, or 2 to 2½ hours after a meal. Don't worry about the time of day; do what works for your family. If the morning is a whirlwind, save it for midday, or maybe the afternoon. You can read about juicing in detail in *Gut and Psychology Syndrome*, Revised and Expanded Edition (pages 303–04).

Be sure to source organic produce, and wash it well. There's no need to peel off any edible skin, since that's where a lot of the good stuff is found. Vegetable juices are lower in sugar and, overall, better detoxifiers. Always add some sort of fat to slow down the absorption of sugars, like egg yolk, cultured cream, avocado, or coconut oil.

Finally, make it fun! Serve your juice in nifty glasses with straws or umbrellas. Let everyone have a turn throwing something into the juicer. If you're using a blender or Vitamix, simply blend 3 to 4 cups produce with 3 cups of filtered water and pour through a fine-mesh strainer. And keep your eyes peeled for a juicer on eBay or craigslist!

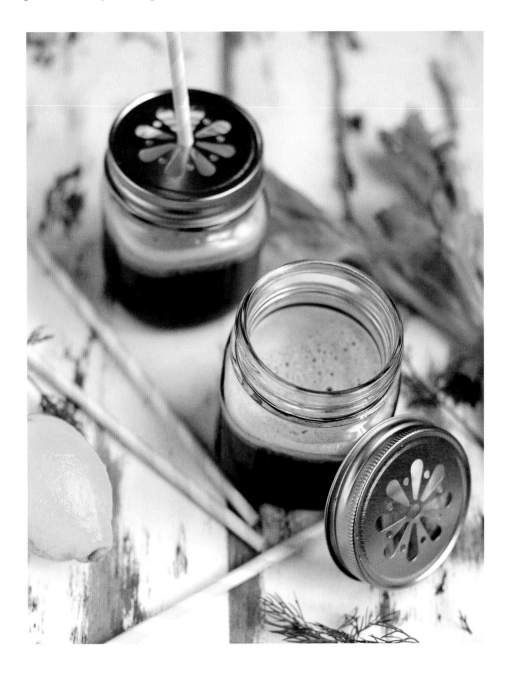

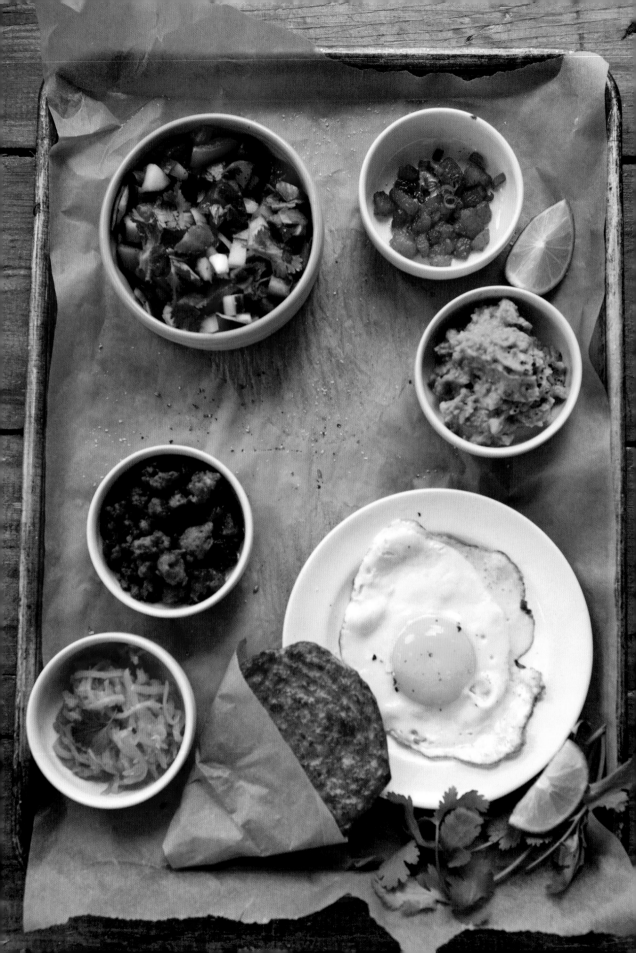

S tage 5 means the introduction of spices—and that means Taco Seasoning. And this stage's soft lettuces and raw vegetables mean Taco Salad. Need I say more? Everyone loves a Taco Salad! Or at the very least, a simple salad with a gorgeous drizzle of olive oil, a squeeze of fresh lemon, and a pinch of sea salt. You can have one with every meal from this point forward. Not to mention the addition of homemade warmed cinnamon applesauce with ghee or coconut oil for a delicious occasional treat. Our kids were over the moon.

With the introduction of seasonings at this stage, you can finally start getting really creative. Now, I am not a professionally trained chef, and I confess that experimenting in the kitchen did not come naturally to me. Initially, I made sure to always use a recipe—I feared screwing things up. But cooking for the GAPS Diet is like on-the-job training, and you earn "head chef" status quickly. Things start to feel easier as you move toward Full GAPS, just up ahead on the horizon. Hopefully you have found a nice rhythm—you have meat stock continuously on the stovetop, often just ladled right into the next pot of soup; kefir (if tolerated) is being turned around every twenty-four hours; your Crock-Pot is familiar and well used in the rotation; mayo and dressings are made every other week; and making ferments is a monthly habit.

However, allow me to cut you some slack. Go ahead and purchase what you don't have time to make, or those foods that you are not yet confident producing. (The resources section will tell you where to purchase things.) But do keep working to master one thing at a time. And let me just say that I have been at this now for nearly six years, and I still make fumbles in the kitchen. And sometimes I still buy the expensive ginger carrots that I know how to make but just can't always find the time. The good news is that it does come together, I promise. You will hit a stride where you are so efficient in the kitchen that nothing goes to waste, and you find yourself banging out several dishes at a time. Leftovers will be incorporated into the next day's menu plan, sometimes even turned into delicious masterpieces. Dinner guests have told me that the previous night's roasted vegetables made a beautiful frittata.

On that note, when you're entertaining or socializing, you may encounter naysayers who fear the fats you have come to know as good friends. Simply hand them a copy of *Put Your Heart in Your Mouth* by Dr. Natasha Campbell-McBride. She wrote this book to challenge the prevailing belief that saturated fat is bad, that eggs give us high cholesterol, that our arteries will clog, and so forth. I refer to it when someone accuses me of starving my kids, or I'm told that I'll be sorry some day when their arteries are so clogged that they drop dead of a heart attack.

Don't worry. These comments will start to roll off your back. I still have to gently remind my mom that my kids' diet now more closely resembles her own mom's diet as a child. Unprocessed, farm-fresh, homemade. And Grean (my grandmother) lived to be ninety-two, despite having smoked for about sixty years of her life and often enjoying her beloved gin with a splash of water. There was not much that Mom could say about that; after all, she wants what's best for them as much as I do. Just stay strong. You are needed as the captain of the ship!

Foods Allowed During Stage 5

Continue with previous stage foods. If you're moving along nicely, and tolerating all foods, you can add raw vegetables and cooked apples. Start with the soft parts of lettuces and peeled cucumber. Once those are tolerated you can slowly add in other raw vegetables. Be sure to cook apples with lots of fat.

In Stage 5, you can add:
- **Spices**
- **Apples** cooked with lots of ghee or coconut oil
- **Raw vegetables:** Start by adding soft lettuces and peeled cucumber; once these are well tolerated, you can add other raw vegetables such as carrots, tomatoes, and onions
- **Fruit as a juice ingredient:** If you tolerate vegetable juice made from carrot, celery, lettuce, and mint, you can start to add small amounts of apple, pineapple, and mango to your juices (avoid citrus fruit at this stage)
- **Pecan flour**

Here are a few Stage 5 juice combinations with a little zip. You can add half a small beet or a carrot to any of these recipes. I often have these on hand but I don't add these for our daughter because she is sensitive to even natural sugars.

Ginger Zing
Serves 1

3 stalks celery	1 lime, peeled
2 cucumbers or 1 English cucumber	1 inch gingerroot
½ pear	Pinch of sea salt, for added minerals

"Green" Apple with a Twist
Serves 1

Small handful greens
½–1 small green apple
2–4 stalks celery

½ lemon, peeled
Pinch of sea salt, for added minerals

Our Go-To Juice
Serves 1

½ head celery
1 English cucumber
1 fennel bulb, with fronds
1 lemon, peeled

1 inch fresh gingerroot (optional)
2 handfuls leafy greens
1 bunch parsley
Pinch of sea salt, for added minerals

Sandy's Regular Juice
Serves 1

My wonderful GAPS practitioner, Sandy Littell, recommended this combination. The beet and carrot are sweet, but they are also nutritious and great for detoxing and flushing out the system. As your body balances and stabilizes, your pancreas will be able to handle a little natural sugar here and there.

A variety of greens (this is the bulk of
   her juice)
2 celery stalks
¼ beet root or beet greens

1 small carrot
1 lemon or lime
Pinch of sea salt, for added minerals

Huevos Rancheros with Cumin Cauliflower Crepes and Crispy Lardo

Traditionally served with beans and corn tortillas, this southwestern dish gets the GAPS treatment with all kinds of delicious meat and vegetable components. Enjoy with Cumin Cauliflower Crepes (recipe follows) and eggs cooked to your liking. Add on whichever sides you wish!

Optional add-ons:
- Fermented Ginger Carrots (page 235)
- Guacamole or chopped avocado (page 116)
- Salsa, either quick homemade or lacto-fermented (page 234)
- Pork sausage (you can also use chicken, beef, or salmon)
- Cilantro
- Lardo (fatback from a pig), cubed and browned in a sauté pan
- Homemade Cultured Cream (page 30)
- Fermented hot sauce, or Hot Nicky (page 241) (Full GAPS)
- When you've built up to handling multiple spices, season your meat with Taco Seasoning (page 128).

Cumin Cauliflower Crepes
Makes 8 crepes

4 eggs
1 teaspoon cumin
1 teaspoon coriander

¼ teaspoon sea salt
1 head cauliflower, riced (instructions below)
1 cup chicken broth

Preheat the oven to 375°F, and line a cookie sheet with parchment paper. Place all of the ingredients in a bowl and mix well. Pour the mixture onto the parchment paper (about ¼ cup per crepe), spreading each one out with the back of a spoon in a small circle (4 to 5 inches in diameter). I can fit three or four per pan. Bake for 10 minutes, or until nicely browned underneath; flip and cook for an additional 5 minutes on the other side.

Variations: The sky's the limit, so get creative! These crepes are versatile and easy to make. For some variety, try cauliflower crepes with:
- Curry or garam masala for an Indian flair (great with Nut Pulp Hummus and vegetables, page 258)
- Garlic and thyme to have alongside a nice salmon or some tuna salad
- Cinnamon with a dollop of honey on top for a delicious breakfast
- Onion and garlic powder for a nice pizza crust

Cauliflower Rice

In your blender, place 1 head cauliflower cut into florets. Fill the blender with filtered water. Turn the blender to high for 3 to 5 seconds. Voilà! You have cauliflower rice. Strain with a fine-mesh strainer. Add cauliflower rice to a pot with 1 cup chicken stock. Simmer, covered, for about 6 minutes. When it is nice and soft, remove from the pan and strain again, making sure it is pretty dry. You can also place it in a tea towel and squeeze out the excess liquid. Save the stock to pour into one of your soups or drink with a spoonful of lard!

Butternut Squash Soup, or "Chicken on Fire"
Serves 6 to 8

They used to call it "Pumpkin Soup" after a children's book. But in the midst of the GAPS Intro, my kids got creative at the table one night. They added piles of shredded chicken and tons of pepper and renamed it "Chicken on Fire"! You never know how you are going to get so much soup into your kids in the beginning of GAPS, so when inspiration (and laughter) strikes, go with it. This is a spiffed-up version of my Butternut Squash Soup in Stage 1.

2 quarts chicken stock to cover (you can supplement with filtered water if you don't have enough stock)

2 tablespoons coconut oil, ghee, or animal fat

2–3 leeks, sliced in half, washed, and sliced again into half-moons (you can substitute 2 onions, chopped)

1 butternut squash, peeled, seeded, and cut into chunks

1 bouquet garni

Sea salt and pepper

2 cups shredded chicken (optional)

Optional Garnishes

Yogurt or cultured cream

Chopped fresh herbs

Soaked and sprouted pumpkin seeds (Full GAPS)

Put the stock and fat in a pot. Add the vegetables and bring to a boil. Reduce the heat to a simmer, add the bouquet garni, and cook, covered, for 30 minutes or until the vegetables are soft and the squash is easily pierced with a fork. Take out the bouquet garni, and remove the soup from the heat. Carefully puree the soup with an immersion blender until smooth. Add salt and pepper to taste along with the chicken, if you like.

Simple Salad with Olive Oil, Lemon, and Sea Salt

Ahhhh . . . the introduction of fresh greens is so welcome! This salad accompanied nearly every meal in our house.

Soft leaf lettuce

Best-quality olive oil

Squeeze of fresh lemon

Pinch of sea salt

Scrumptious Chicken in a Crock-Pot
Serves 6 to 8

Spices are a wonderful addition to Stage 5. Feel free to use any chicken parts on the bone. If you don't have time for the spices, just add onions, salt, pepper, and fat and turn it on! This is a great way to enjoy a tougher chicken. Often the soy-free pastured chickens you get from your farmer are not as plump as what you might find in the grocery store. This meat will just fall off the bone!

2 teaspoons paprika

1 teaspoon sea salt

1 teaspoon onion powder

1 teaspoon dried thyme

½ teaspoon garlic powder

1 teaspoon curry powder

1 teaspoon dried basil

1 teaspoon dried sage

¼ teaspoon black pepper

2 onions, sliced

1 whole chicken

Animal fat or ghee

Combine the dried spices in a small bowl. Place the onions in the bottom of the slow cooker. Remove any giblets from the chicken, wash it, and pat it dry. Rub the spice mixture all over it. You can even put some of the spices inside the cavity and under the skin covering the breasts. Rub some fat over the chicken. Put the prepared chicken on top of the onions in the slow cooker, breast-side down, cover it, and turn it on to high. There is no need to add any liquid. Cook for 3 to 4 hours on high or 6 to 8 on low (for a 3- to 4-pound chicken), or until the meat is falling off the bone. Don't forget to make your homemade broth to freeze for Full GAPS right in the Crock-Pot with leftover bones, a few feet, a head, celery, carrot, and onion.

Squash Popovers
Makes 4 popovers

These make a great breakfast as well as a delicious dessert.

2 tablespoons ghee or coconut oil
1 cup butternut squash puree (page 70)

8 large eggs
¾ teaspoon sea salt

Optional Flavorings

½ cup finely shredded coconut, 1
    teaspoon cinnamon, and 1 apple,
    chopped

½ cup cooked ground sausage and ¼ cup
    chopped fresh herbs

Preheat the oven to 350°F. Place 1 to 2 teaspoons of melted fat in each of your "popover" cups. (You can also use mugs or ovenproof ramekins.) Blend the squash with eggs until well mixed. For a sweeter popover, add the coconut, apples, and cinnamon, and blend again. Or for a savory version, try the cooked ground sausage with fresh herbs. Fill the popover cups halfway full with batter. Bake in the oven for 30 minutes, or until the popovers have "popped"!

Cooked Apples
Serves 6 to 8

This is delicious and curbs any sweet tooth for kids craving a treat after or between meals. By mixing in loads of added fat, you will slow the absorption of sugar and create a more nutritious and satisfying treat.

12 organic apples, peeled, cored, and
    sliced (leave skin on in Stage 6)

1 tablespoon cinnamon (optional)
¼–⅓ cup ghee or coconut oil

Cook the apples in a pan with a few inches of filtered water until soft (25 to 30 minutes). Leave as is or blend with your immersion blender. Add the cinnamon and fat, and serve warm. Delicious with a dollop of cultured cream (page 30) and an added dash of cinnamon. Kids love to add their own toppings!

Fermented Pear and Apple Chutney
Makes 1 pint

This is a great recipe I learned from Scott Grzybek, of Zukay Live, at the Weston A. Price conference. It is delicious with Roasted Pork Sausage with Red Onion and Butternut Squash (page 190).

2 pears	Pinch of allspice
2 apples	Pinch of cardamom
1 teaspoon sea salt	Small handful raisins
1 teaspoon cinnamon	

Chop the pears and apples into chunks, and place in the food processor. Process until you reach your desired consistency (I prefer this a little chunky). Add the remaining ingredients, and pulse a few more times to incorporate. Place in a pint-sized mason jar, cap tightly, and leave on the counter to ferment for 3 days. Store in the fridge.

Beef Jerky
Serves 4 to 6

I suggest making more of this than you think you need. It doesn't last long!

Jerky is one of those foods I once thought sounded too complicated. I'd been dragging my feet to make it. Then I purchased my first quarter of a cow from friends Willie and Cecile of Two Sisters Farm in Warren, Maine, and it was time to get serious about different cuts of meat and learning how to use them. Cecile generously dropped off an amazing book called *Good Meat* by Deborah Krasner, and I devoured its pages. I highly recommend trying this recipe, adapted from Krasner's original. It's very easy, no dehydrator required, and my kids and husband gobble it up every time I make it. It's great for school lunches and snacks on the go. Feel free to leave out the cayenne; it's delicious with or without.

½–1 pound grass-fed beef (top round or sirloin tip roast)	1 teaspoon kelp or dulse (great for added minerals and flavor)
¼ cup coconut aminos	½ teaspoon ground chipotle
2 tablespoons filtered water	½ teaspoon freshly ground black pepper
1 garlic clove, pressed	¼ teaspoon sea salt
1 teaspoon chili powder	¼ teaspoon cayenne

Take your meat out of the freezer and let it thaw to the point of partially frozen. It is much easier to cut in this state. Slice the meat ⅛ inch thick and as long as you can make it. In a medium glass bowl, mix together the coconut aminos, water, garlic, chili powder, kelp, chipotle, black pepper, salt, and cayenne. Add the meat and mix thoroughly. Cover the bowl with plastic wrap, and let it marinate in the fridge overnight.

Heat the oven to 175°F. Line a baking sheet or two with parchment paper, or place a cookie rack on top of a cookie sheet. Place your beef jerky on a plate lined with paper towels or cloth to absorb some of the marinade. Wipe off the excess garlic. Line the slices on the baking sheet in rows. Slow-roast the meat for 3 hours, then turn it over and slow-roast for 1 to 2 more hours. This can be refrigerated for up to 3 weeks . . . if it's not gobbled up sooner!

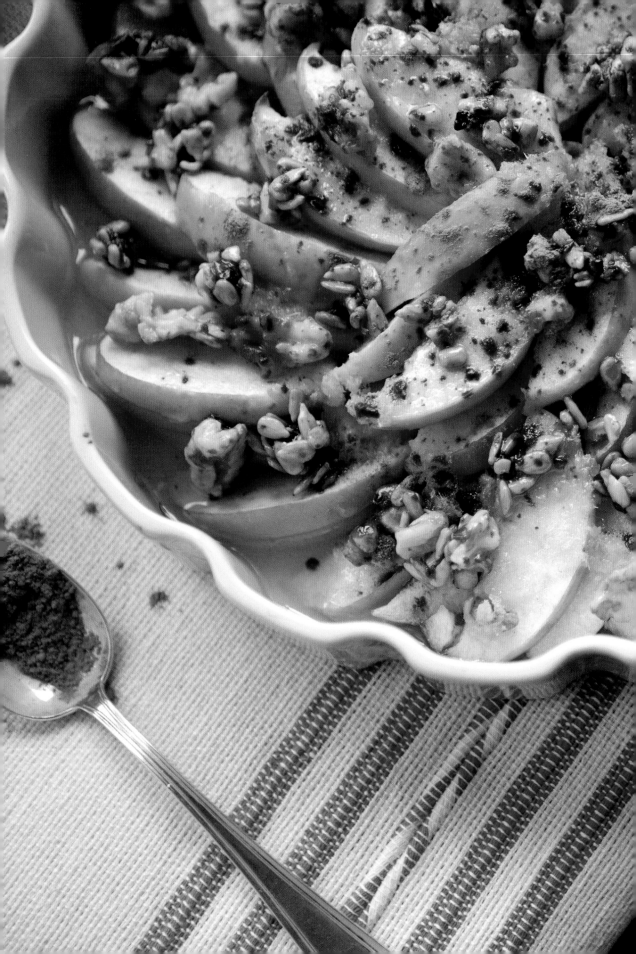

The countdown is officially here, and you should be eating a pretty "normal" diet at this point. Well, I suppose it wouldn't seem normal to a person coming directly from the Standard American Diet, but hopefully GAPS will become your new normal very shortly. People on GAPS are often amazed to look back at their old eating habits. When I remember my days of fat-free eating, I can't believe I ever even thought that was normal, let alone healthy. Now if someone tells me that fat makes you fat, I tell them about my husband, who dropped thirty pounds in about thirty days while drinking coconut oil in his tea and putting a tablespoon of pastured lard in his soup three times a day.

It's true: You will lose weight in the beginning, especially if you have weight to lose. I, too, lost weight and had a few comments that I was looking too skinny, but I knew that the GAPS program is a very balancing diet, and that things would soon even out. Sure enough, I eventually put some weight back on and landed right where I should be. Nick has maintained his weight loss and gets comments almost daily on how great he looks. Our kids, too, remain happy, strong, and healthy looking.

Unlike fat, overindulgence in sweets *can* make you fat. And most important: It's sugar that fuels the proliferation of bad bacteria in our guts. So be mindful of this as you enter Stage 6, which features the introduction of GAPS-friendly desserts and an increase in honey if desired and tolerated. The introduction of these desserts is not necessary for healing; it's an option since there's always a time and place for a sweet treat in everyone's life.

Many of the GAPS-approved treats are nut-based. Nuts are very high in calories, so be sure to keep them to a limit; it is easy to overdo it! I have tried to keep desserts fairly simple in our lives, such as seasonal fruit with cultured cream or Coconut Manna. I always add fat to modulate sugar absorption. Fruit and honey still break down into sugar in the body, so just because bananas and mangoes are now GAPS-legal doesn't mean you should have three a day! Try to keep fruit consumption to about 1/2 cup per day, if that, and go with a seasonal option whenever possible since it's more nutritious, ecological, and delicious. Remember: You don't want your taste buds getting hijacked again by those pesky bad bacteria clamoring for sugar down there, but every now and then something special is called for. So just be mindful, keep it limited, have fun, and enjoy that treat when you have one!

Foods Allowed During Stage 6

Continue with previous stage foods. If everything you have introduced thus far is well tolerated, slowly introduce some raw peeled apple as well as other raw fruits, introducing one at a time. Raw honey can be increased, as can GAPS-friendly desserts. If possible, use dried fruit, instead of honey, as the sweetener for cooked desserts.

In Stage 6, you can add:

- **Raw fruits:** Gradually introduce raw fruits from GAPS-approved list of fruits: pears, kiwis, huckleberries, raspberries, nectarines, apricots, berries (all kinds), blackberries, very ripe bananas (covered with brown spots), blueberries, coconut, cherries, prunes, peaches, and ugli fruit
- **Honey:** You can increase honey if it's tolerated
- **Brazil nuts:** Introduce these slowly, and watch for tolerance issues
- Additional foods: raisins, cinnamon, coriander, coconut milk, dates, black radishes, and capers
- **Sweet treats and baked goods:** Gradually introduce these as allowed on the diet

---

Cinnamon Apple Bake
Serves 6 to 8

7–10 apples (depending on size of baking dish), cut in quarters and sliced into half-moons

¼ cup coconut oil, plus 1 tablespoon for topping

2 tablespoons ghee, plus 1 tablespoon for topping (use additional coconut oil if you cannot tolerate ghee)

2 inches fresh gingerroot, peeled and grated

2 tablespoons honey, plus 1 tablespoon for topping

¼ teaspoon sea salt

½ cup sprouted walnuts, chopped

½ cup sprouted sunflower seeds

Preheat the oven to 350°F. Spread the apple slices in a spiral in a round ovenproof dish. In a small saucepan, melt the coconut oil and ghee together over medium-low heat. Add the grated ginger and 2 tablespoons honey, then pour the mixture over the apples. Sprinkle with sea salt, and bake for 20 minutes. While the apples bake, place the walnuts and sunflower seeds in a saucepan with the reserved coconut oil, honey, and ghee. Cook ever so lightly for about 5 minutes. Remove the apples from the oven, and pour the nut mixture over them, making sure to coat them all evenly with the oils. Enjoy as is, or with a dollop of cultured cream (page 30).

Coconut Macaroons
Makes 10 to 12 macaroons

2 cups unsweetened shredded coconut
6 egg whites
¼ cup raisins
2 teaspoons Homemade Vanilla Extract
  (page 96)

Pinch of sea salt
3–4 dates, pitted, soaked, and
  blended (optional)
1 tablespoon raw cacao powder for
  chocolate macaroons (optional, Full GAPS)

Preheat the oven to 350°F. In a bowl, combine all of the ingredients. Line a baking sheet with parchment paper, and place 1 tablespoon of dough for each cookie on the sheet. Press down to flatten each cookie out a bit. Bake for 12 to 15 minutes until golden. After you've made mayonnaise (page 107), this is a great way to use up leftover egg whites. (See photo on page 265.)

Variation: For a sweeter macaroon add dates to the recipe and follow these instructions: Remove the pits, and soak the dates in a bowl of hot filtered water for 5 minutes (if you don't have the time for this step, skip it). Add the dates to your food processor with all the remaining ingredients except the raisins. Process to combine and form a sticky dough. If it is too dry, add a teaspoon or two of the date water. Fold in the raisins, and follow the cooking instructions above.

Lemon Curd
Serves 4 to 6

After making macaroons, this is a great way to use up the leftover egg yolks! This is surely a crowd pleaser!

6 egg yolks
Juice and zest of 3 lemons
¼ cup of honey

¼ cup ghee or butter, chilled (Full GAPS)
Pinch of sea salt

Using a double boiler, whisk together the egg yolks, lemon juice, lemon zest, and honey, combining thoroughly. Slowly whisk in small pieces of the ghee or butter (if you're using it) until it's all incorporated. Gently simmer, and occasionally whisk the mixture until it thickens, 5 to 10 minutes. Once you have reached the desired custard-like consistency, remove the curd from the heat and place it in a bowl of ice-cold water to halt the cooking process. Pour it into a glass dish or single-serving ramekins, and store in the fridge. Yum!

Power Smoothie
Serves 2 to 4

My amazing homeopath friend, Joette Calabrese from Homeopathy Works (see resources), inspired this delicious and nutrient-dense smoothie. Her CD *Secret Spoonfuls* is all about getting the good stuff into your kids.

1 quart 24-hour cultured, raw yogurt
   or kefir
½ cup raw cultured cream
1–2 tablespoons extra-virgin coconut oil
   (melted at a low temperature) or
   2 tablespoons coconut manna
   (if tolerated)
1–3 raw pastured egg yolks (from a reliable source, such as a local farmer)

1–2 tablespoons raw honey
1 teaspoon cold-pressed flax oil, or fresh
   ground flax (Full GAPS)
1 banana, ½ cup combined raspberries,
   strawberries, and/or frozen fruit
1 teaspoon vanilla extract (optional;
   homemade recipe below)

Place all of the ingredients in a blender, and blend until smooth. Be sure to crack your eggs in a bowl before transferring to the blender, just in case you ever happen to get a rotten egg.

Homemade Vanilla Extract
Makes 1 pint

According to Joette, vanilla supports thyroid function and is a great addition to any smoothie once tolerated.

8–10 highest-quality vanilla beans

1 pint organic, or best-quality, vodka, rum,
   or brandy

Score the beans down the center to release the flavor. Place them in a pint-sized bottle (I love to use Grolsch bottles; see resources). Fill the bottle with alcohol, cap, and let it sit in a cool, dark place for 1 month or so. Upon finishing the vanilla, you can reuse the beans one more time: Just fill the bottle up with alcohol again, and repeat the steeping process. This is a great cost savings and makes a lovely housewarming gift!

The Benefits of Smoothie Ingredients

Joette Calabrese, HMC, CCH, RSHom(Na)

- Raw cultured cream: fat-soluble vitamins such as B_6 and valuable enzymes
- Raw yogurt (or kefir): probiotics that provide live enzymes necessary for quality digestion
- Pastured raw egg yolks: omega 3 fatty acids and cholesterol needed for mental development; fat-soluble vitamins A and D
- Coconut oil: nourishing fat that is loaded with antibacterial, antifungal, and antiviral properties and promotes brain development and strong bones
- Raw honey: enzymes that aid in digestion and ward off infections
- Flax oil: unsaturated omega 3 fatty acids that support lungs, brain, and skin

Fruit "Jell-O"
Serves 4 to 6

2 pints hot filtered water
1 tablespoon raw honey (optional)
2 tablespoons gelatin (I like Great Lakes Gelatin unflavored)

½–1 cup fresh or frozen berries (pomegranate seeds and blueberries are some of our favorites)

Bring the water to a boil, then separate it into two bowls and let it cool slightly. Dissolve the honey in one bowl and the gelatin in the other. Stir the gelatin, and let it set for about 10 minutes. Add the two together and stir. Pour into a glass dish, Jell-O mold, or fun glasses, then add the berries or your flavorings of choice (see the variations below). Stick it in the fridge to set overnight or until completely gelled. You can eat the "Jell-O" out of the dish—but if you carefully pop it out and onto a plate, the berries will be right on top! We always top with a dollop of cultured cream (page 30).

Variations: Try these flavor combos:
- Lemon or lime zest and coconut flakes
- Blueberry "Jell-O" with a dollop of cultured cream on top
- Kombucha with fruit, water kefir with fresh lemon juice, or fruit kvass of any kind (if you're using live cultures, be sure to not add to very hot water)

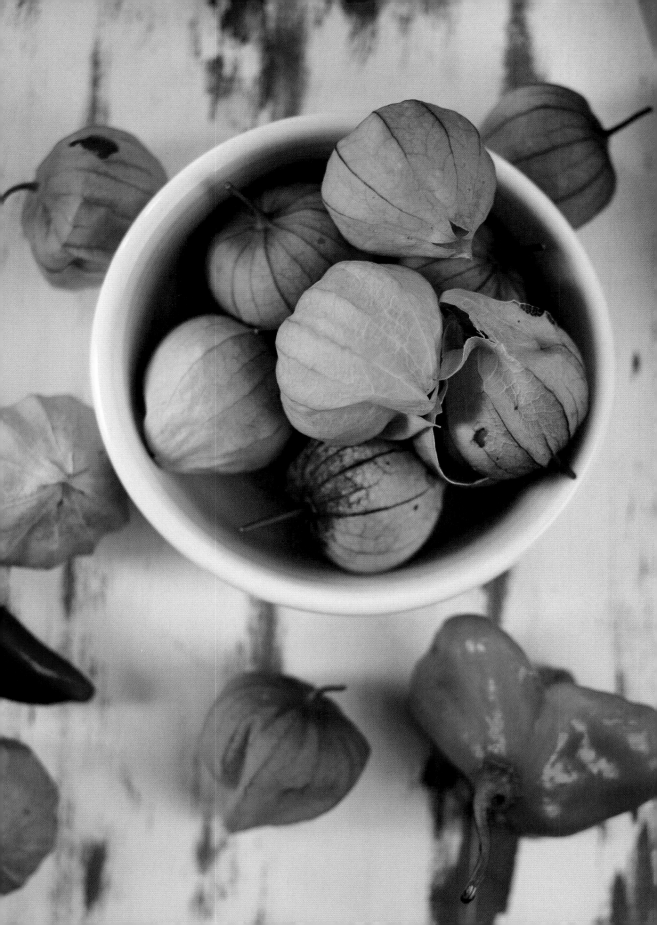

The Full GAPS Diet

You made it! You have graduated to Full GAPS. Congrats! I know that was quite a whirlwind experience, and—although well worth the effort—very challenging. But you did it, and now you're ready. Much healing has occurred over the past weeks, and you are ready for a little more flexibility and variety, so it's time to spread your wings and get more creative in the kitchen. Remember that you have "head chef" status by now: You're like a GAPS pro, pumping out stock, picking carcasses, rotating ferments, and serving up three nutritious meals a day! Pat yourself on the back, again and again. Don't get discouraged if there are setbacks: An unexpected emergency, an infection, and even vacations are all situations that could derail you somewhat. Just pick yourself up by the bootstraps and return to the Intro Diet for a week or longer if necessary. At this point you have the tools, so take the reins and do what you have to do.

Once you have successfully moved through the stages of the GAPS Intro, and you have no digestive issues or other concerns, you can go ahead and move to the Full GAPS Diet. Please read carefully the section on the Full GAPS Diet in *Gut and Psychology Syndrome*, Revised and Expanded Edition (pages 152–54) and refer to page 100 on "Foods Allowed on the Full GAPS Diet" and page 103 for "Foods Not Allowed." Otherwise, you are now free to roam the book. Peruse the recipes and see what jumps out at you. Many of them will be familiar to you, but with a healthier, healing twist. Remember that every body is different, and if you experience symptomatic setbacks such as hand flapping, bloating, trips to the bathroom, and hyperactivity, be sure to stop, breathe, evaluate, and then go with your gut. Take note of what you ate that day, or the few days prior, and remove the offender for another three to five days before trying again. Diversify your diet slowly and deliberately.

The Full GAPS Diet should be followed for a minimum of two years. I know, I know . . . Even good old Nick still says to this day, "There is no way we are staying on this diet for two years." But I just keep plugging away in the hope that his desire for a Bud and some pizza will eventually disappear. Remember that you are in charge of your body only, and letting go of some control when you can't bend other people's will is okay. It's their journey, too, and there's only so much you can do. Concentrate on healing yourself and those who need it most. If some participants in your family have lesser symptoms, they may be able to introduce non-GAPS foods after a year.

At this point I am sure you have seen positive changes. Remember, this is no overnight fix, there will be ups and downs, and you will survive! Keep the faith and keep your eyes on the prize! Bravo, my friends, bravo!

Foods Allowed on the Full GAPS Diet

Adapted from *Gut and Psychology Syndrome*, Revised and Expanded Edition by Dr. Natasha Campbell-McBride, pages 159–63 ("Recommended Foods").

- Almonds, including almond butter and oil
- Apples
- Apricots, fresh or dried
- Artichoke, French
- Asiago cheese
- Asparagus
- Aubergine (eggplant)
- Avocados, including avocado oil
- Bananas (ripe only with brown spots on skin)
- Beans, dried white (navy), string beans, lima, split peas, haricots
- Beef, fresh or frozen
- Beets or beetroot
- Bell peppers (green, yellow, red, and orange)
- Berries, all kinds
- Black radish
- Blue cheese
- Bok choy
- Brie cheese
- Broccoli
- Broth, homemade, made from bones of poultry, beef, lamb, pork, and fish
- Brussels sprouts
- Butter
- Cabbage
- Camembert cheese
- Canned fish, in olive oil or water only
- Capers
- Carrots
- Cashew nuts, fresh only
- Cauliflower
- Cayenne pepper
- Celeriac
- Celery
- Cellulose in supplements
- Cheddar cheese
- Cherimoya (custard apple)
- Cherries
- Chicken, fresh or frozen
- Cinnamon
- Citric acid
- Coconut, fresh or dried without sweetener or additives
- Coconut milk
- Coconut oil
- Coffee, weak and freshly made, not instant
- Colby cheese
- Collard greens
- Coriander, fresh or dried
- Cream, cultured, homemade from raw cream
- Cucumber
- Dates, fresh or dried, additive-free
- Dill, fresh or dried
- Duck, fresh or frozen
- Edam cheese
- Eggplant (aubergine)
- Eggs, fresh
- Filberts (hazelnuts)
- Fish, fresh, frozen, canned in its juice or oil
- Game, fresh or frozen
- Garlic
- Ghee, homemade
- Gin, occasionally
- Gingerroot, fresh
- Goose, fresh or frozen
- Gorgonzola cheese

- Gouda cheese
- Grapefruit
- Grapes
- Havarti cheese
- Herbal teas
- Herbs, fresh or dried, additive-free
- Honey, raw
- Juices freshly pressed from permitted fruit and vegetables
- Kale
- Kefir, homemade from raw milk
- Kiwi fruit
- Kumquats
- Lamb, fresh or frozen
- Lemons
- Lentils
- Lettuce, all kinds
- Lima beans, dried and fresh
- Limburger cheese
- Limes
- Mangoes
- Meats, fresh or frozen
- Melons
- Monterey Jack cheese
- Muenster cheese
- Mushrooms
- Mustard, without any non-allowed ingredients
- Nectarines
- Nut flour or ground nuts
- Nutmeg
- Nuts, all kinds fresh, properly soaked and dried
- Olive oil, virgin cold-pressed
- Olives, without any non-allowed ingredients
- Onions
- Oranges
- Papayas
- Parmesan cheese
- Parsley
- Peaches
- Peanut butter, without additives
- Peanuts, soaked and dried, roasted
- Pears
- Peas, dried split and fresh green
- Pecans
- Pepper, all kinds
- Pheasant, fresh or frozen
- Pickles, without sugar or any other non-allowed ingredients
- Pigeon, fresh or frozen
- Pineapples, fresh
- Pork, fresh or frozen
- Port du Salut cheese
- Poultry, fresh or frozen
- Probiotic (lacto-fermented) foods using all allowed vegetables
- Prunes, dried without any additives
- Pumpkin
- Quail, fresh or frozen
- Raisins
- Rhubarb
- Romano cheese
- Roquefort cheese
- Rutabagas
- Satsumas
- Scotch, occasionally
- Seaweed, fresh and dried
- Shellfish, fresh or frozen
- Spices, single and pure without any additives
- Spinach
- Squash (summer and winter)
- Stilton cheese
- Stock, homemade, made from bones of poultry, beef, lamb, pork, and fish
- String beans
- Swiss cheese
- Tangerines
- Tea, weak and freshly made, not instant

- Tomato juice, without additives except salt
- Tomato puree, pure without any additives except salt
- Tomatoes
- Turkey, fresh or frozen
- Turnips
- Uncreamed cottage cheese (dry curd)

- Vinegar: apple cider, white, rice, and coconut
- Vodka, very occasionally
- Walnuts
- Watercress
- Wine, dry, red or white
- Yogurt, homemade from raw milk
- Zucchini

Where Are the Beans?

You might have noticed that beans and legumes are excluded from the recipes in this book. That's because I haven't yet introduced beans and legumes to our family's repertoire of GAPS recipes. For this collection, I've focused on creating recipes that my family could also enjoy. This is not to say that you can't try adding them back into your diet when you are ready; just be sure to follow proper legume soaking and prep procedures. For more information, see *Gut and Psychology Syndrome*, Revised and Expanded Edition by Dr. Natasha Campbell-McBride, pages 137–38.

Foods Not Allowed on the Full GAPS Diet

Adapted from *Gut and Psychology Syndrome*, Revised and Expanded Edition by Dr. Natasha Campbell-McBride, pages 164–67 ("Foods to Avoid").

- Acesulfame
- Acidophilus milk
- Agar-agar
- Agave syrup
- Algae
- Aloe vera (once digestive symptoms are gone, you can introduce it)
- Amaranth
- Apple juice
- Arrowroot
- Artificial sweeteners: Nutrasweet, Splenda, Equal, etc.
- Aspartame
- Astragalus
- Baked beans
- Baker's yeast
- Baking powder and raising agents of all kinds apart from pure bicarbonate of soda (see note at the Coconut Butter Bread recipe, page 118)
- Balsamic vinegar
- Barley
- Bean flour and sprouts
- Bee pollen
- Beer
- Bitter gourd
- Black-eyed peas
- Bologna
- Bouillon cubes or granules
- Brandy
- Buckwheat
- Bulgur
- Burdock root
- Butter beans
- Buttermilk
- Canned vegetables and fruit
- Cannellini beans
- Carageenan
- Carob
- Cellulose gum
- Cereals, including all breakfast cereals
- Cheeses, processed, and cheese spreads
- Chestnut flour
- Chèvre cheese
- Chewing gum
- Chickory root
- Chickpeas
- Chocolate
- Cocoa powder (see note at the "Nutella" recipe, page 262)
- Coffee, instant and coffee substitutes
- Cooking oils
- Cordials
- Corn
- Corn syrup
- Cornstarch
- Cottage cheese
- Cottonseed
- Couscous
- Cream
- Cream cheese
- Cream of tartar
- Dextrose
- Drinks, soft
- Fava beans
- Feta cheese
- Fish, preserved, smoked, salted, breaded, canned with sauces
- Flour, made out of grains
- FOS (fructo-oligosaccharides)
- Fructose

- Fruit, canned or preserved
- Garbanzo beans
- Gjetost cheese
- Grains, all
- Gruyère cheese
- Ham
- Hot dogs
- Ice cream, commercial
- Jams and jellies
- Jerusalem artichoke
- Ketchup, commercial
- Lactose
- Liqueurs
- Margarines and butter replacements
- Meats, processed, preserved, smoked, and salted
- Millet
- Milk: animal, soy, rice, canned coconut milk
- Milk, dried
- Molasses
- Mozzarella cheese
- Mung beans
- Neufchâtel cheese
- Nuts, coated or commercially prepared
- Oats
- Okra
- Parsnips
- Pasta of any kind
- Pectin
- Postum
- Potato, sweet and white
- Primost cheese
- Quinoa
- Rice
- Ricotta
- Rye
- Saccharin
- Sago
- Semolina
- Sherry
- Soda (soft drinks)
- Sour cream, commercial
- Soy
- Spelt
- Starch
- Sugar or sucrose of any kind
- Tapioca
- Tea, instant
- Triticale
- Turkey loaf
- Vegetables, canned or preserved
- Wheat and wheat germ
- Whey powder or liquid
- Yacon syrup
- Yams
- Yogurt, commercial

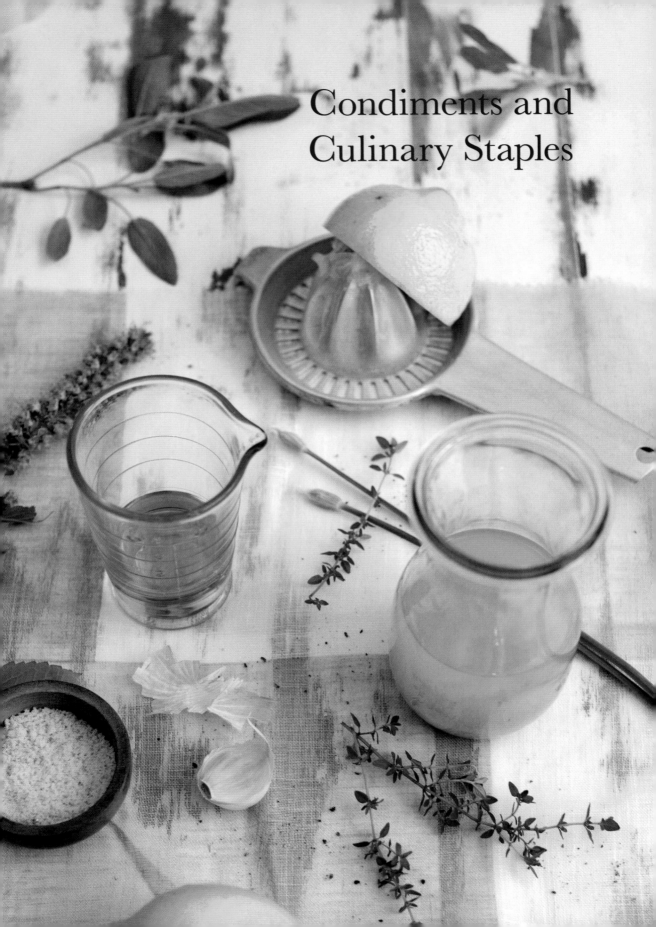

Condiments and Culinary Staples

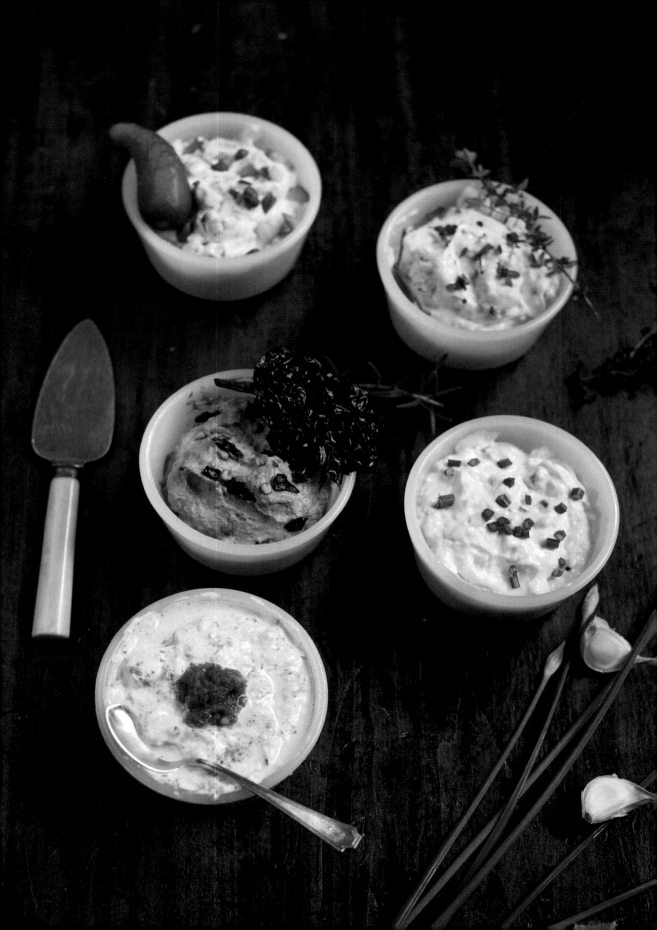

MAYO: OUR FAVORITE CONDIMENT
Makes 1½ cups

At the very beginning of our GAPS journey, it was Nick's and my turn to host a monthly supper club. We were a bit nervous, to say the least, what with our new diet and alcohol restrictions. It went great, though: We served burgers, sides, and a big salad with a variety of ferments. But at the last minute, I realized we were out of ketchup—oops! Bring on the mayo and garlic aioli! We ended up going through a double batch that night, and the next day I was inundated with emails requesting the recipe. Turned out that everyone loved our GAPS-approved meal! If you have added whey or pickle juice, it will help your mayo last longer while adding enzymes and increasing the nutrient content. After making mayonnaise, leave it out, well covered, on the counter for 7 hours before refrigerating. It will keep for up to 2 months in your fridge.

3 pastured egg yolks
1 teaspoon dried mustard
Juice of ½ small lemon
½ teaspoon sea salt
½ cup extra-virgin coconut oil
½ cup quality olive oil
⅛ cup whey, sauerkraut juice, or
  pickle juice (optional)

In a food processor, pulse to mix the yolks, mustard, lemon juice, and salt. Melt the coconut oil just slightly so that it becomes liquid. (If you heat it too high, it will start to cook the eggs.) Add to olive oil. Then, with your food processor on, *slowly* pour in the oil mixture until it emulsifies; start with 1 to 2 drops, then a few more, then a few more, then begin a slow, steady stream. My good friend Talie tipped me off, in one of my cooking classes, that the Cuisinart actually has a little tiny hole in the top attachment piece for streaming in oils. This makes making mayo a lot easier! Add whey, briefly blend until incorporated. Using a rubber spatula, put the mayo in a jar and keep in the fridge. Use within a week.

GARLIC AIOLI
Makes 1½ cups

This stuff is the bomb! Use the same instructions as above, adding garlic into food processor with yolks, mustard, lemon juice, and salt.

3 pastured egg yolks
1 teaspoon dried mustard
3 cloves garlic
Juice of ½ small lemon
½ teaspoon sea salt

½ cup extra-virgin coconut oil
½ cup quality olive oil
2 tablespoons whey, sauerkraut juice, or
    pickle juice (optional)

Mayo and Aioli Mix-Ins

These combos make great dressings, dips, or sandwich spreads; try them blended into your egg or chicken salad!

- Minced shallots and herbs
- Minced red pepper, garlic, and cilantro
- Chopped scallions
- Seeded and chopped red chile peppers
- Jalapeño, garlic, cilantro, lime zest (orange works well, too), cumin, and chili powder
- Garlic, chives, parsley, and tarragon
- Chipotles in adobo, lime, roasted garlic, sea salt, and pepper
- Dijon mustard, honey, chopped chives, mustard seeds, and Hot Nicky (page 241)
- "Tartar sauce": aioli with chopped fermented pickles or capers, and diced red onion
- Hot Nicky Mayo: A few tablespoons added to about 1 cup of mayo is a staple in our house (page 241)

LACTO-FERMENTED MUSTARD TWO WAYS

Yellow Mustard
Makes roughly 1 pint

¾ cup mustard powder
½ cup organic, raw apple cider vinegar
  or coconut vinegar
2 tablespoons whey or pickle juice
1 teaspoon sea salt
1½ tablespoons lemon juice
¼ teaspoon organic turmeric
½ teaspoon garlic powder
¼ teaspoon paprika

Thoroughly mix all of the ingredients and transfer to a pint-sized mason jar. Cover tightly, and leave on the counter at room temperature for 3 days, then refrigerate. Yellow Mustard will last several months refrigerated.

Fermented Whole Grain Honey Mustard
Makes roughly 1 pint

This recipe is inspired from Cultures for Health, a wonderful website offering loads of information, recipes, and resources on culturing foods. This is great with Caesar salad (see Caesar Dressing, page 128).

¾ cup pickle juice or whey
¼ cup whole yellow mustard seeds
¼ cup whole brown mustard seeds
  (these are hotter than the yellow)
1 small shallot, minced
1 clove garlic, minced
1 tablespoon honey (optional)
1 teaspoon sea salt

In a bowl, combine the pickle juice, mustard seeds, shallot, and garlic, and let sit overnight. In a food processor, mix the mustard seed combination with the honey (if you're using it) and salt. Continue to blend until you reach the desired consistency. Transfer to a pint-sized mason jar, cover tightly, and leave on the counter for 3 days. Honey Mustard will last several months refrigerated.

LACTO-FERMENTED HOMEMADE KETCHUP
Makes 1 pint

I searched and searched for a good ketchup recipe that my kids would love. After playing around, I discovered that this one is magic. It's especially delicious on burgers, with homemade mayo and mustard. Bingo!

14 ounces organic tomato paste
  (no salt added)
⅓ cup fermented pickle juice or whey
2 tablespoons apple cider vinegar
¼ teaspoon mustard powder
⅛ teaspoon ground cloves
⅛ teaspoon ground allspice
⅛ teaspoon cayenne
½ teaspoon sea salt
2–4 tablespoons honey

Whisk all of the ingredients together in a bowl. Pour the ketchup into a mason jar. Cap and leave at room temperature for 2 days, then move to the fridge. This will last several months.

LACTO-FERMENTED BBQ SAUCE
Makes 1 pint

This is delicious with the Pork Carnitas (page 183).

1 onion, finely minced
2 cloves garlic, pressed
1 cup tomato paste
¼ cup honey
2 tablespoons apple cider vinegar
2 tablespoons coconut aminos
½ teaspoon sea salt
1 teaspoon paprika
¼ teaspoon cinnamon
½ teaspoon chili powder
1 teaspoon dry mustard
Pinch of cayenne
2 tablespoons sauerkraut juice, pickle
  juice, or whey

Place all of the ingredients in a pint-sized mason jar, and cap with a lid. Leave on the counter for 2 days before placing in the fridge.

CHIMICHURRI
Makes approximately 1 pint

1 bunch flat-leaf parsley, stems removed
1 bunch fresh cilantro, stems removed
¼ cup fresh oregano, stems removed (optional)
¼ cup roughly chopped red onion
4–6 cloves garlic
1 teaspoon sea salt
½ teaspoon freshly ground black pepper
1 tablespoon apple cider vinegar or coconut vinegar
Juice of 1 lime
¾ cup unrefined extra-virgin olive oil

In a food processor, pulse together the parsley, cilantro, oregano, onion, and garlic. Add the sea salt, pepper, vinegar, and lime, and pulse a few more times to blend well. Empty the herb mixture into a bowl and stir in the olive oil. Serve by the spoonful over steak, burgers, sausages, or chicken. Fresh and wonderful!

HOLLANDAISE SAUCE
Makes approximately 1 cup

We always had broccoli, asparagus, and artichokes with hollandaise when I was a kid. It sure was an effective way to get me to eat my vegetables. I loved them all!

3 farm-fresh egg yolks
½ cup sea salted butter
Juice of 1 lemon

Place all of the ingredients in a double boiler over medium heat and whisk constantly for about 5 minutes. Make sure to keep taking the mixture off the heat if you think it's going to curdle. You can serve this at room temperature.

BÉARNAISE SAUCE
Makes approximately 1 cup

I always tease my husband and say, "Would you like some steak with your béarnaise?" After adopting the Nourishing Traditions diet, he was thrilled to know that it was actually a nutritious indulgence! His mother makes it every year at Christmastime, and she shared with me this trick for sauce that accidentally scrambles or curdles: Add a few drops of water and keep whisking off the heat, until the curdles disappear. It should turn back to a nice smooth sauce.

This recipe is from *Nourishing Traditions* by Sally Fallon Morell; it makes about 1¼ cups. We always double it!

2 tablespoons finely chopped shallots
1 tablespoon finely chopped fresh
   tarragon, or 1 teaspoon dried tarragon
1 tablespoon dry white wine
2 tablespoons white wine vinegar
5 egg yolks at room temperature
½ cup butter, preferably raw, cut
   into pieces
Fresh lemon juice
Pinch of sea salt
Pinch of pepper

In a small saucepan, combine the shallots, tarragon, wine, and vinegar. Bring to a boil and reduce to about 1 tablespoon of liquid. Strain into a medium-sized, heatproof bowl or pot (or you can pour it all in to keep the shallots and tarragon in the sauce). In another bowl, beat the egg yolks with a whisk. Now create a double boiler by setting the bowl containing your vinegar reduction over a pan of simmering water, Add about half the butter, piece by piece, to the liquid, whisking constantly until melted. Then add the egg yolks very slowly, drop by drop, or in a very thin stream, whisking constantly. Add the remaining butter, and whisk until well emulsified. The sauce should now be warmed and slightly thickened. Remove from the heat, and whisk in lemon juice, sea salt, and pepper to taste. May be kept warm in a bowl set over hot water. Whisk occasionally until you're ready to serve.

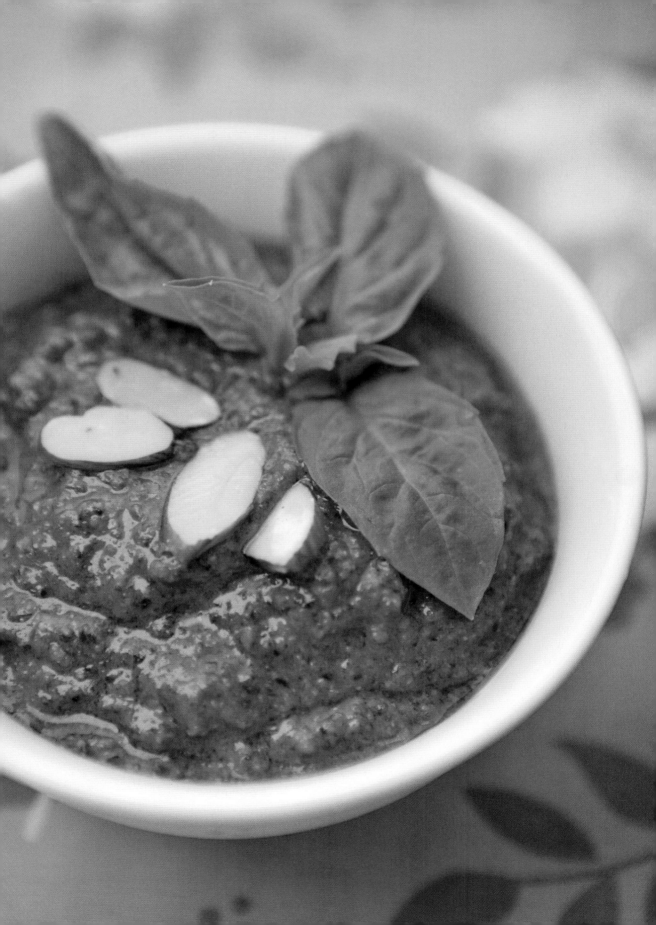

PESTO SEVEN WAYS

Special thanks to Laura at First Root Farm for inspiring the creative pesto combinations listed below. Follow the "Classic Basil" instructions for them all.

Classic Basil
Makes approximately 1 pint

2–4 cups fresh basil
½ cup olive oil
½ cup grated raw Parmesan (optional)
½ cup pine nuts
2 cloves garlic for every cup basil leaves
Zest and juice of 1 lemon
Sea salt and pepper

Combine all of the ingredients in a food processor or Vitamix (you'll need a tamper) or food processor, and pulse or blend until well combined; you may need to add a little olive oil to get it going. While the machine is running, slowly drizzle in the olive oil until your desired consistency is achieved. Season with salt and pepper to taste. Put in a pint-sized mason jar, and store in the fridge.

Cilantro Pesto
Makes approximately 1 pint

1–2 bunches fresh cilantro
¼ cup olive oil
5 cloves garlic
2–3 tablespoons lemon juice

Sea salt and freshly ground pepper
1 teaspoon fresh grated ginger (optional,
　 but recommended!)

Mellow Fennel
Makes approximately 1 pint

1–2 bulbs fennel, chopped and lightly
　 sautéed in coconut or olive oil until soft
　 (about 10 minutes)
½ cup olive oil

5 cloves garlic
½ cup lightly toasted walnuts
Sea salt and pepper

Smoky Sage
Makes approximately 1 pint

1 cup sage leaves, packed
¼ cup olive oil
5 cloves garlic

1–2 tablespoons lemon juice
Sea salt and pepper
Nuts if you wish (pine nuts are nice)

Lemon Dill
Makes approximately 1 pint

1 bunch fresh dill
4–5 cloves garlic
¼ cup olive oil
1–3 tablespoons lemon juice

Sea salt and pepper
Grated lemon zest for a lovely color and
    extra lemony flavor

Zesty Arugula
Makes approximately 1 pint

1–2 bunches arugula, washed and
    trimmed (young and tender is more
    mellow; older is spicier)
¼ cup olive oil (walnut oil would
    be nice, too)
½ cup walnuts

¼ cup grated Parmesan (optional)
3–5 tablespoons fresh lemon juice
Sea salt and pepper
3 cloves garlic, optional (for a
    super-spicy batch!)

Sun-Dried Tomato Pesto
Makes approximately 1 pint

4 cups fresh basil
½ cup pine nuts
10–15 sun-dried tomatoes (packed in
    olive oil, or dried and reconstituted
    with filtered water)

2–3 garlic cloves
1 cup olive oil
Sea salt and pepper

GUACAMOLE
Makes 1 to 2 cups

One of our favorite accompaniments to any meal.

2 ripe avocados, mashed
Juice of 1 lime
Pinch of sea salt
1 tomato, chopped (optional)
½ bunch fresh cilantro,
  chopped (optional)

Mix all of the ingredients together and serve. This is a great source of healthy fat for the kids, and it will keep them satiated longer. This is almost a daily staple in our house.

ED GIOBBI'S SWEET MARINARA SAUCE
Serves 4 to 6

I learned this delicious recipe at a preserving class taught by Ed's daughter, Eugenia Bone. I have modified it a bit for GAPS. It freezes beautifully, so consider busting out your biggest stockpot in order to double or triple the quantities! Enjoy it over roasted vegetables, spaghetti squash, chicken, or just as is.

3 tablespoons ghee, butter, or
  preferred fat, divided
1 medium onion, diced (about 1 cup)
2 medium carrots, chopped (about 1 cup)
2 large cloves garlic, minced
4 cups fresh tomatoes, chopped; or
  2 jars or cans (28 ounces each)
1 tablespoon chopped fresh basil
1 teaspoon dried oregano
Sea salt and freshly ground black pepper

Heat 1 tablespoon of the ghee, butter, or preferred fat in a large saucepan over medium heat. Sauté the onion, carrots, and garlic until soft, about 10 minutes. Add the tomatoes and cook for 15 minutes, until the sauce is bubbling. Then reduce the heat to a simmer. For a smooth sauce, zap with an immersion blender. Throw in the herbs, season with salt and pepper, then cook for another 15 minutes. Finally, add the remaining 2 tablespoons fat and stir until melted.

ROASTED TOMATO SAUCE
Makes 2 to 3 quarts

If you ever get a bumper crop of tomatoes, make and freeze this recipe. You will enjoy a flavorful burst of summer during the cold winter months! Try this sauce over boneless chicken thighs; top them with a blend of cheeses, bake at 350°F for 45 minutes . . . and presto! A quick "Chicken Parm" that everyone will love. If you want to preserve the raw enzymes in the cheese, just grate it on top upon removing it from the oven.

25 fresh tomatoes, quartered
8 onions, quartered
10 cloves garlic, smashed
2 handfuls fresh herbs, chopped
¼ cup ghee, lard, or coconut oil, melted
Sea salt and pepper

Preheat the oven to 450°F. In a large roasting pan, mix the tomatoes, onions, garlic, and herbs with the melted fat. Season generously with sea salt and pepper. Roast for 30 minutes, gently stir, then cook for another 30 minutes. Leave as a chunky sauce, or zap with the immersion blender for a smooth one.

COCONUT BUTTER BREAD
Makes 1 loaf

I'd been making bread with coconut flour but felt conflicted, knowing that it had a significant amount of fiber in it, which can be irritating to the gut. Also, I really don't like cooking my nut flours. So I asked my wonderful GAPS practitioner, Sandy, and she recommended this great recipe from lovingourguts.com: It gives you the benefits of the fat with the fiber when using coconut butter. She informed me that baking soda is not acceptable on its own but should be okay when incorporated into recipes in small amounts. It has a much better consistency than the other bread I had tried. It works for sandwiches as well as burger buns and egg sandwiches. (I always double it!) It's best sliced and toasted.

1 cup coconut butter
5 eggs, at room temperature
¼ cup coconut oil or pastured lard
½ teaspoon sea salt
¾ teaspoon baking soda

Preheat the oven to 300°F. Grease a 5 by 9-inch loaf pan and place the jar of coconut manna into a pan of simmering water to soften it. This will take about 10 to 20 minutes. Stir the coconut butter to make it consistent throughout. Put all of the ingredients into a bowl, and mix with a handheld blender. Be sure to blend enough so that there are no lumps at all. The consistency should be like cake batter. Pour the batter into the loaf pan and bake for 40 to 50 minutes. Let it cool for 10 minutes. Store in the fridge. (Do not send this off to school right out of the oven in an airtight container: It may come back uneaten and moldy. Once it's cooled in the fridge, though, it's good to go.)

Variation: For cinnamon raisin bread, fold in 1 teaspoon cinnamon and ¼ cup raisins, pour into the loaf pan, and follow the instructions above.

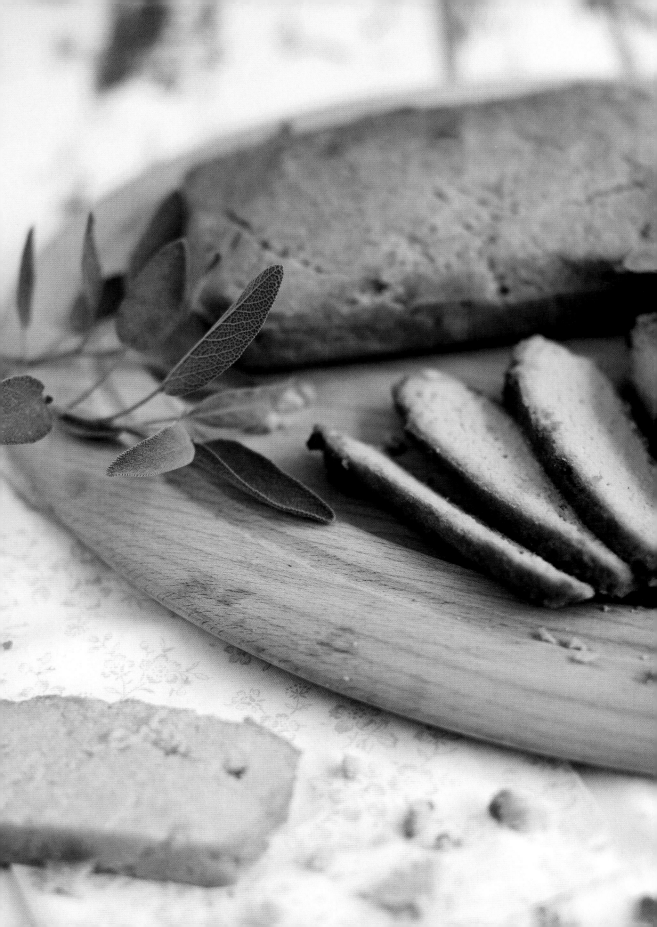

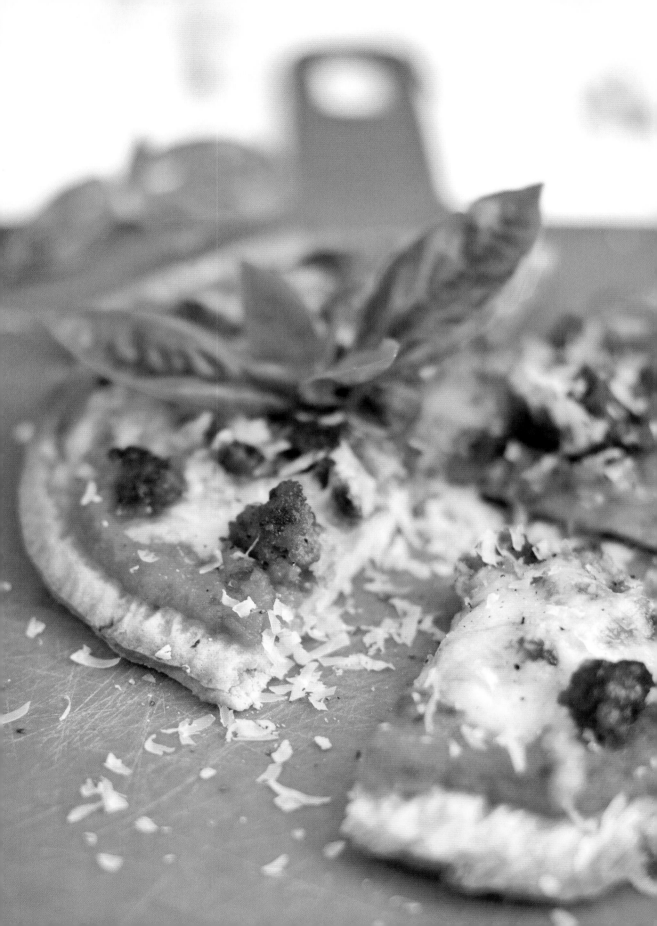

COCONUT FLOUR PIZZA CRUST
Makes 4 crusts

This is a great savior for birthday parties and special occasions. Store-bought coconut flour is very high in fiber and can be hard on damaged guts, which is why it is not GAPS-compliant. Homemade coconut flour is much lighter and fluffier; it isn't as dense or high in fiber as store-bought, so you shouldn't have issues with your gut. However, start slowly and see how you handle it. Increase as tolerated.

¾ cup homemade coconut flour
½ cup coconut oil or lard
6 pastured eggs
1 teaspoon sea salt
1 teaspoon garlic powder
1 cup Ed Giobbi's Marinara Sauce (page 116) (or sauce of choice); you can also use tomato paste and herbs
½–1 cup shredded cheese

Preheat the oven to 350°F. Place all of the ingredients (except the sauce and cheese) in a bowl and mix with a hand mixer until there are no lumps. On a parchment-lined cookie sheet, spread out the dough in 4- to 5-inch circles using the back of a spoon. Bake for 10 minutes, flip, and bake for another 5 to 10 minutes. Add the marinara sauce and cheese and pop back in the oven for another 5 minutes. Let cool slightly, cut, and serve.

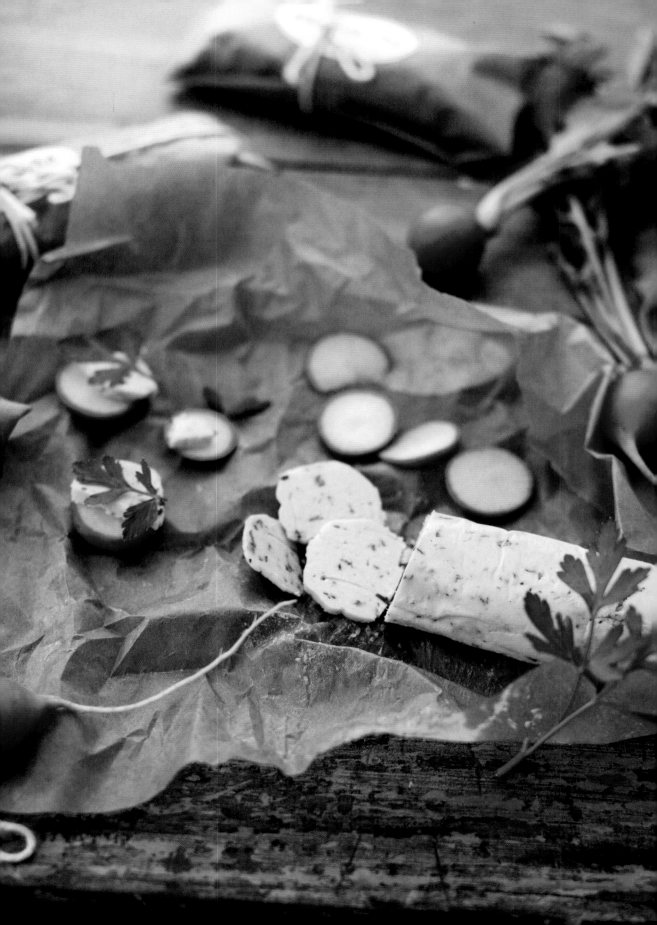

HERBED BUTTER
Makes ½ cup

This make-ahead condiment is easy, delicious, and nutritious. A great way to get some extra fat into your kids, Herbed Butter (also called compound butter) can be made with nearly any type of flavoring you choose. We all miss a nice piece of bread and butter, so try one of the following recipes with some Coconut Butter Bread (page 118) and enjoy! Raw, cultured butter (page 31) is best because of its nutritional and probiotic benefits; but really, any good grass-fed butter is still great! My go-to grocery store butter is unsalted Kerry Gold from Trader Joe's.

Be sure to start with very soft butter. Leave it out on the counter for a few hours or overnight, and let it come to room temperature. This makes incorporating the ingredients easier. Flavorings are blended into the softened butter with a rubber spatula. Always add a pinch of sea salt! Place your blended butter on a piece of parchment, and roll it into a log. Fold it over and fasten the ends, label, and refrigerate or freeze.

Fresh Herb Butter

Terrific on burgers, steak, roast beef, roast turkey, chicken (rub under the skin before cooking), fresh fish, and vegetables, roasted or raw:

½ cup unsalted butter
1 tablespoon minced sage
1 tablespoon minced thyme
1 tablespoon minced rosemary

2 cloves fresh garlic, pressed
Pinch of sea salt and fresh
   cracked pepper

Honey Ginger Cumin Butter

Delicious over fish, chicken, roasted carrots, or cauliflower.

½ cup unsalted cultured butter
1 teaspoon raw honey
Zest of 1 lime
½ teaspoon cumin
¼ teaspoon ground ginger

1 teaspoon cinnamon
1 teaspoon chopped fresh thyme
Black sesame seeds
Pinch of sea salt

Vanilla Cinnamon Honey Butter

Scrumptious on bread, crackers, apples, pancakes, or an open-faced nut butter and butter sandwich.

½ cup unsalted butter
Scrapings of 1 vanilla bean
1 teaspoon raw honey

1 teaspoon cinnamon
Pinch of sea salt

Chili Lime Butter

This is fabulous on flank steak or with huevos rancheros pancakes.

½ cup unsalted butter
1 chile, finely diced (seeded, optional)
Zest of 1 lime
Juice of ½ lime

1 shallot
2 tablespoons chopped fresh cilantro
Pinch of sea salt

Other Combinations

- Cilantro, cumin, and curry
- Blue cheese or Gorgonzola
- Chopped sun-dried tomatoes (in olive oil) and basil
- Chive, mustard, and shallot
- Parsley, shallots, garlic, and lemon zest
- Coconut, date, cinnamon

Note: *Don't forget to add a pinch of sea salt.*

Dressings

When I first saw Sally Fallon Morell speak at a Weston A. Price conference, she started her lecture by saying, "Salads are killing America." I sat there thinking, *What the heck—now salads are bad for us? What's next?* Well, at the end of her lecture she concluded by saying it's the dressings we dump all over our salads that are killing us. These dressings are typically filled with rancid vegetable oils (like canola and soybean oil) and even high-fructose corn syrup. Way to ruin a salad!

If you are eating salads, do yourself a favor and stick to healthy oils: olive oil and expeller-pressed flax oil. Most of the vitamins in our vegetables are fat-soluble, so adding a dressing full of healthy fats better enables our bodies to absorb the nutrients. Making your own dressing might seem like one more thing that you don't have time to do, but I promise that it's easy, plus you can double or triple your batch to store in the fridge for a few weeks. Plus, making your own is a real money saver, too. Just remember to set it out a bit before mealtime to allow the oils to come to room temperature for easier pouring.

Salad Dressing Basics
Monica Corrado, MA, CNC, traditional food and GAPS chef

Dressings may be categorized into three types:
- Oil and vinegar (vinaigrette)
- Cream or cheese
- Puree

For a basic vinaigrette dressing: This dressing is the basis or the foundation of the other dressings. Once you know this formula, you can make any of the others simply by adding cream, cheese, what have you. All of the recipes are written in "parts." Remember that a "part" can be an ounce or ¼ cup. Just use the same unit of measurement throughout the recipe.

1 part any vinegar (apple cider, coconut, or white wine) or citrus juice

3 parts good-quality olive oil (or 4 parts if you prefer more oil)

1 forkful, roughly ½ tablespoon, mustard (fermented is best), or best store-bought organic mustard you can find

1 T expeller-pressed flax oil

Then add garlic or ginger, and any herbs you like.

For a cream dressing, add 2 parts cultured cream, sour cream, yogurt, or kefir to the basic recipe. For a cheese dressing, add 2 parts Roquefort, blue, or another cheese.

For a puree, add 2 parts tahini and celery, onion, and carrots, or a handful of an herb you like, such as fresh basil.

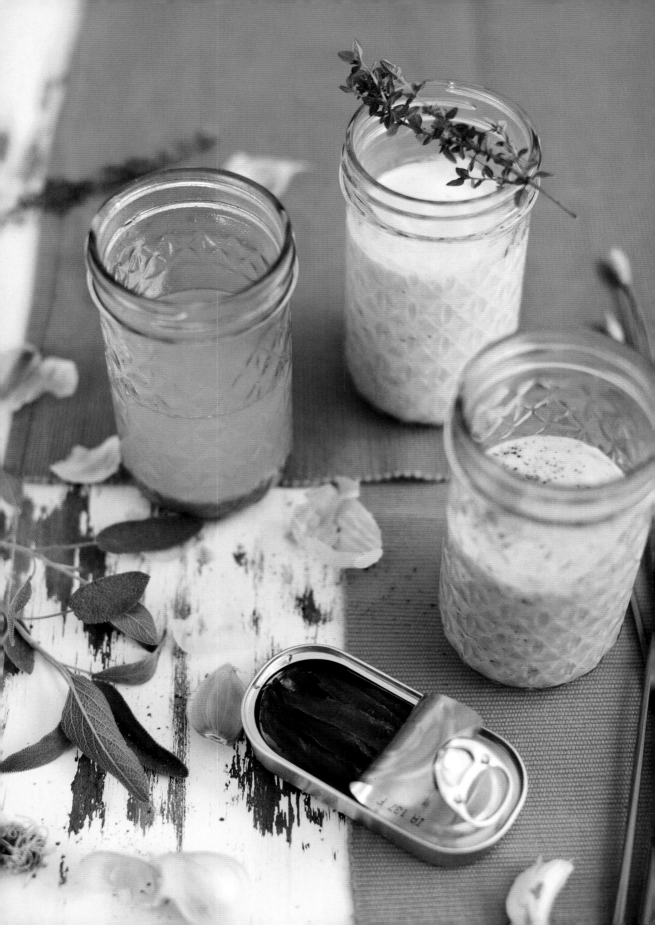

You will have fun concocting your own recipes, but in the meantime, here are a few for inspiration.

CULTURED CREAM AND KEFIR HERB DRESSING/DIP
Makes 1 cup

½ cup raw kefir
½ cup raw cultured cream
2 tablespoons chopped fresh herbs
Zest of 1 lemon
Juice of ½ lemon
½ teaspoon sea salt
Fresh cracked pepper

Place the ingredients in a bowl and whisk together. You can also assemble the ingredients in a jar and shake them to combine for easy storage.

BASIC VINAIGRETTE
Makes 1 cup

1 teaspoon organic mustard (I like stone-ground or lacto-fermented even better; page 109)
½ teaspoon sea salt
1 clove garlic, pressed (optional)
Freshly cracked pepper
Fresh chopped herbs (optional)
3 tablespoons lemon juice, fresh-squeezed orange juice, or raw apple cider vinegar
¾ cup olive oil

Place the mustard, seasonings, and lemon juice in a bowl and whisk together. Slowly stream in the olive oil while whisking to emulsify. Store in a clean glass mason jar in the fridge.

CAESAR DRESSING
Makes approximately 1 pint

This will make a salad lover out of almost any kid!

2 tablespoons lemon juice

4–6 cloves garlic, minced

1 tablespoon stone-ground mustard

2 tablespoons homemade mayonnaise

½ cup extra-virgin olive oil

1 cup grated Parmesan (optional)

1 small jar anchovy fillets, minced
   (optional)

½ teaspoon sea salt

Freshly ground black pepper

Blend together the lemon juice, garlic, mustard, and mayonnaise. Slowly stream in the olive oil and finish off with freshly grated Parmesan cheese, minced anchovies, and salt and pepper to taste. Alternatively, put all of the ingredients in a mason jar and use an immersion blender to blend.

TACO SEASONING
Makes 1 cup

A few years back, my friend Kristin had dinner with the wonderful ladies from Nourish MD. I scoured their awesome website, and this has been a staple that my kids make for me monthly ever since. I order the spices in bulk, and I usually triple the recipe!

2 tablespoons chili powder

5 teaspoons sweet paprika

4 teaspoons ground cumin

1 tablespoon onion powder

2 teaspoons sea salt

2½ teaspoons garlic powder

⅛ teaspoon cayenne pepper

Combine all of the ingredients and store in an airtight container for up to a year.

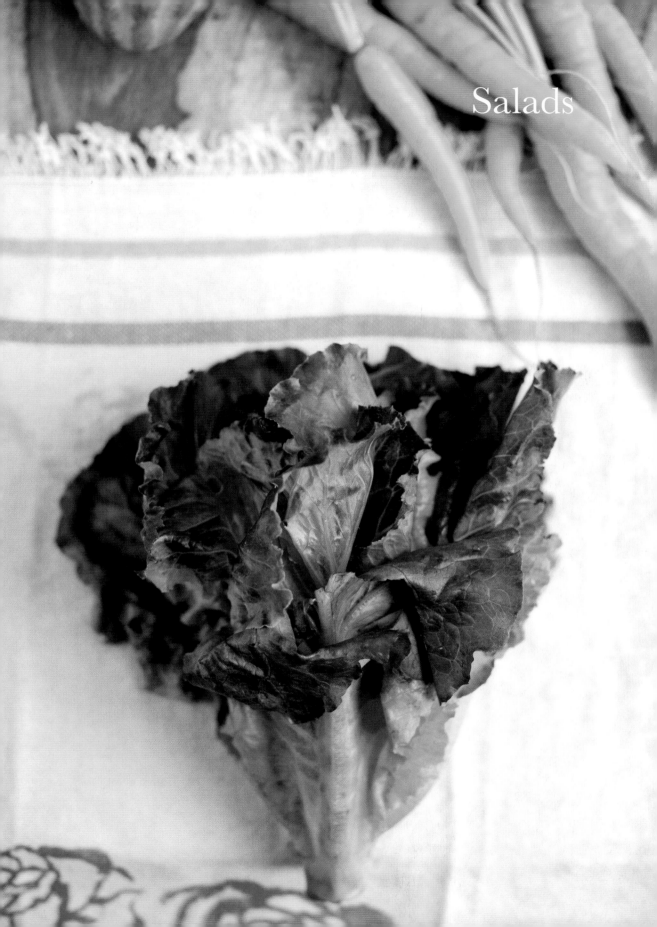

Salads

CAULIFLOWER "COUSCOUS"
Serves 6 to 8

This quick and easy salad is a wonderful accompaniment to many entrées. You could also have it for lunch with chicken or fish on top. And it makes a delicious hot side when tossed with roasted vegetables, herbs, olive oil, sea salt, and fresh cracked pepper.

1 head cauliflower, grated or riced
   (page 87) (about 4 cups)
4 cups filtered water
Juice of 1 lemon
Zest of 2 lemons
2–3 tablespoons olive oil
½ bunch flat-leaf parsley, chopped
½ cup pistachios
½ red onion, sliced
5 dates, cut into small pieces
2 handfuls fresh arugula
½ teaspoon sea salt
Fresh black pepper

To rice the cauliflower, place the florets in a Vitamix, add the water, and blend on high for 5 to 10 seconds. Strain through a fine-mesh colander, pressing out any excess water with the back of a spoon. (You can also use a food processor fitted with the grater or S attachment. No water necessary.)

Tip the riced cauliflower into a bowl, add remaining ingredients, toss, and serve.

If you don't want your cauliflower raw, you can also steam it for about 6 minutes, or simmer it briefly in chicken stock, then strain well. Let it chill before adding the remaining ingredients.

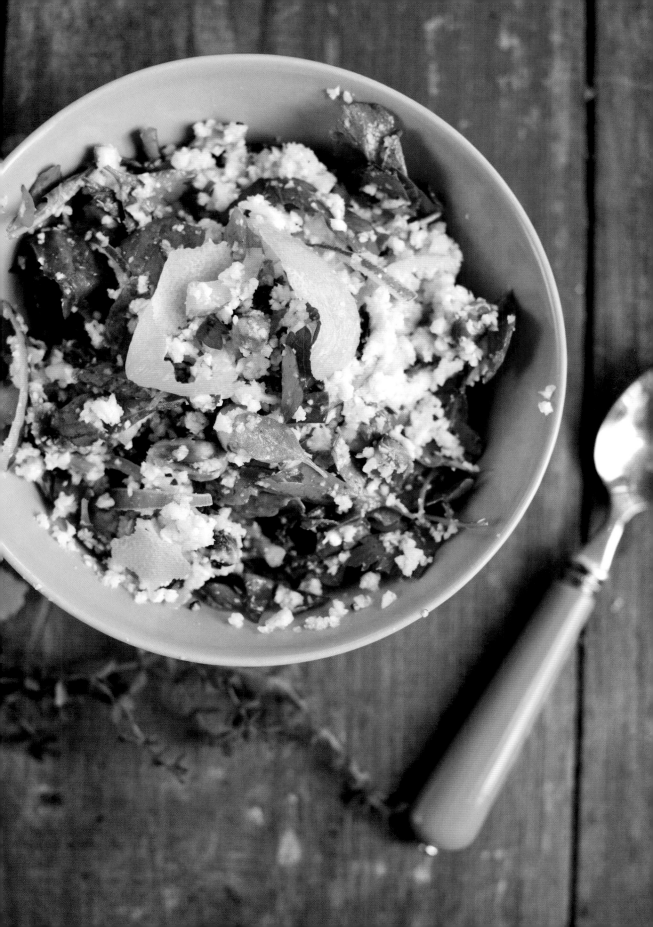

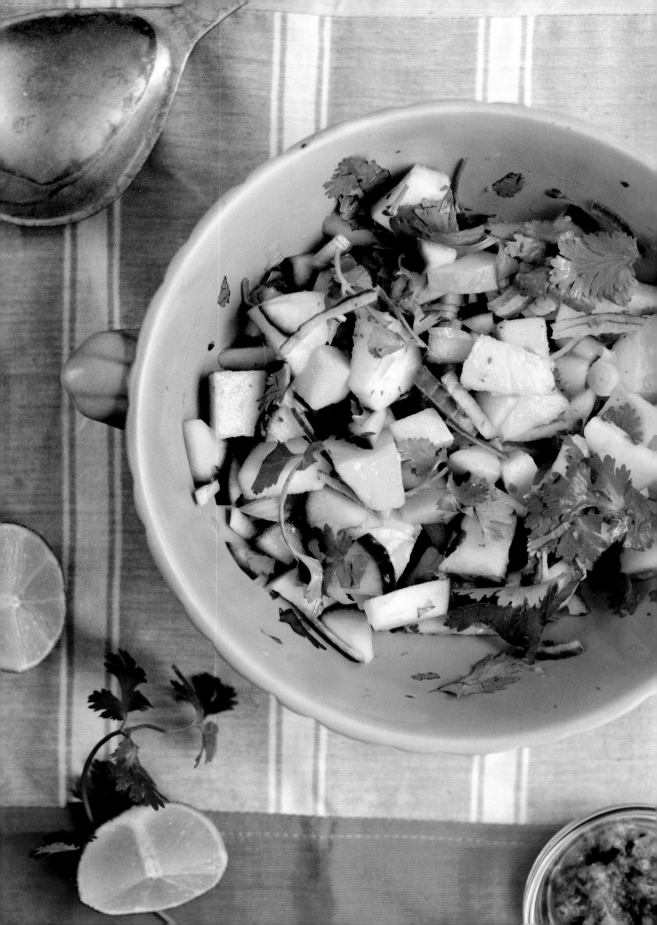

CARIBBEAN CHOW SALAD
Serves 6 to 8

My beloved former babysitter Carleen and her family from Trinidad introduced me to this refreshing summer salad. The sweetness and spiciness will make your taste buds sing. It's a beautiful side for any tropical or Mexican dish!

1 apple, diced
1 mango, peeled and cubed
½ bunch scallions, diced
½ cucumber, peeled, seeded, and
   cut into half rounds
½ onion, red or white (red is prettier)
3 cloves garlic, minced or pressed
Juice of ½ lime
Handful of chopped cilantro
Sea salt and pepper

Mix all of the ingredients together in a bowl. If you want to spice it up, add half a spoonful of Hot Nicky (or more to taste; page 241).

RAW KALE SALAD
Serves 4 to 6

I am very fortunate to have an awesome health food store right in my neighborhood. In fact, I often say that The Natural Gourmet, in West Concord, has changed my life! Its patient and generous staff has guided my family's transition to healthy eating. Remember, when you enter such a specialty shop the employees are passionate about what they're doing. Ask for recipes and advice when you need to; most people are eager to share their knowledge.

One of The Natural Gourmet's top-selling prepared foods is their Raw Kale Salad, which inspired this recipe. Raw kale is not something we should eat every day, as it can be harsh on a compromised digestive tract, but once in a while it's a tasty and beautiful use of the nutrient-dense greens.

1 head curly or lacinato kale
2 tablespoons olive oil
Juice of 1 lemon
1 tablespoon apple cider vinegar
¼ cup crispy pumpkin seeds
½ red onion, thinly sliced
1 avocado, diced
Sea salt and pepper

Tear off the kale leaves and discard the stems. Chop into bite-sized pieces, and toss in a bowl with the olive oil. Massage the kale for 5 minutes to help break down some of the rigid plant cell structure, which can be irritating to the gut when eaten raw. (This also helps diminish the bitterness and toughness.) The greens will wilt a bit and turn a darker green. Adjust your acidity with a squeeze of lemon, sprinkle with your add-ons, and you are all set. No real dressing is required. This will stay fresh in the fridge for a few days, and it will get easier to digest the longer it marinates.

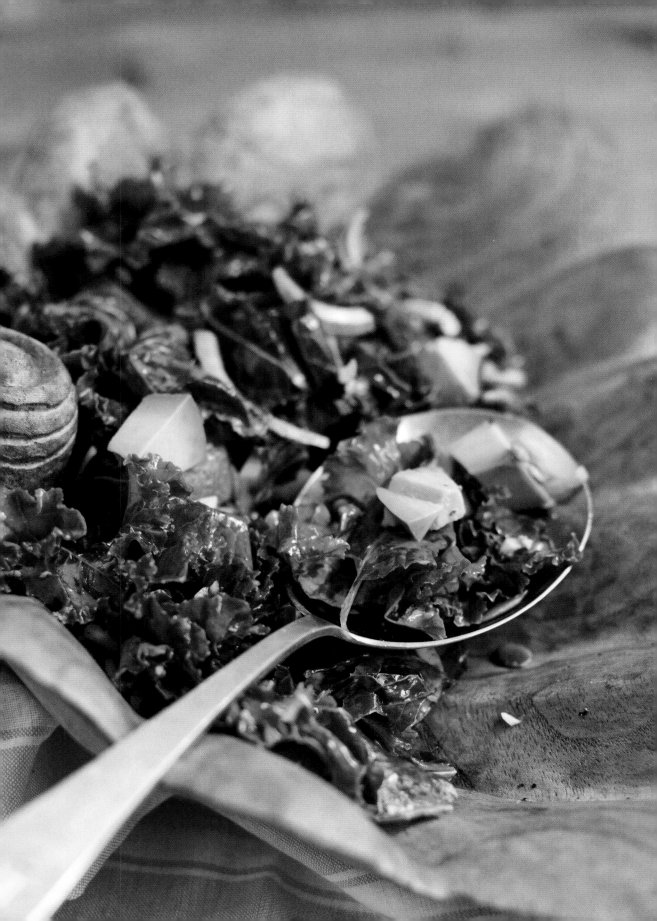

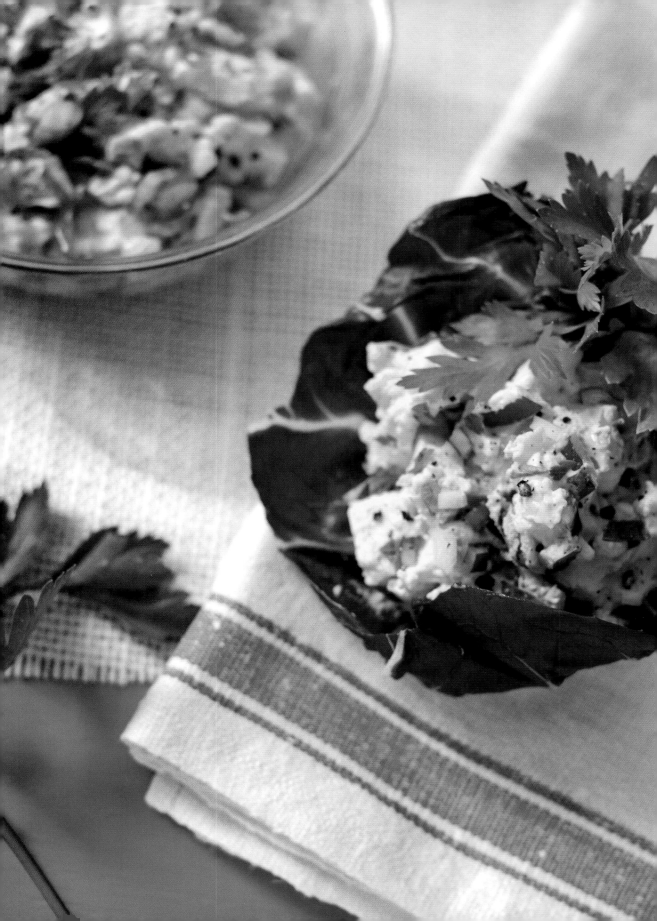

LUNCH SALADS:
CHICKEN, TUNA, EGG, OR SALMON

When time is of the essence (which it usually is in our house), I am psyched to have these salads in the fridge. I just go for some fresh greens on the side with Onion Bread (page 246), Flax Crackers (page 248), or Sweet Crackers (page 245) and a serving of fermented vegetables. For all of the salads below, simply toss the ingredients together in a bowl and mix well.

Chicken Salad
Serves 4 to 6

1 pound cooked chicken breast, shredded or cubed (Poached Chicken, page 44, is wonderful in this recipe)
3 tablespoons homemade mayonnaise or Garlic Aioli (pages 107 and 108)
½ bunch flat-leaf parsley or 2 tablespoons chopped fresh tarragon
¼ red onion, diced
2 celery stalks, diced
Sea salt and pepper

Salmon Salad
Serves 2 to 4

1 5–6 oz can wild-caught salmon (I love Vital Choice) or leftover cooked salmon fillet
2 tablespoons homemade mayonnaise or Garlic Aioli (pages 107 and 108))
½ red onion, diced
Juice of ½ lemon
½ bunch parsley
1 tablespoon chopped fresh dill (optional)
1 tablespoon capers (optional)
Sea salt and pepper

Tuna Salad
Serves 2 to 4

I used to buy tuna in olive oil, but my GAPS practitioner Sandy made a great point that the olive oil industry can be a bit corrupt and mix olive oil with undesirable and unhealthy oils (like soybean oil) to save money. I now buy tuna in water and add olive oil or mayonnaise myself. Our daughter enjoys tuna with olive oil, because her egg allergy keeps her from having the mayo. It is delicious either way.

1 5–6 oz jar or can wild-caught tuna in olive oil
2 tablespoons homemade mayonnaise or Garlic Aioli (pages 107 and 108), or olive oil
½ red onion, diced

Juice of ½ lemon
1 small handful fresh parsley, chopped
Salt and pepper
1 tablespoon capers (optional)
1 tablespoon fresh dill, chopped (optional)

Egg Salad
Serves 2 to 4

6 hard-boiled eggs (page 68)
2 tablespoons homemade mayonnaise or Garlic Aioli (pages 107 and 108))
½ bunch flat-leaf parsley
¼ red onion, diced fine

1 fermented pickle, chopped (optional)
1–2 tablespoons chopped fresh dill (optional)
Sea salt and pepper

THAI CHICKEN SALAD WITH A KICK
Serves 6 to 8

This salad is flexible. Feel free to use whatever vegetables you have on hand; it is the dressing that really ties it all together. If you are staying away from raw cabbage, then substitute another lettuce you love. Radicchio, arugula, mizuna—oh my!

Sea salt and pepper
2 whole chicken breasts (I like bone-in skin-on breasts, but you can use any chicken pieces you wish)
2 tablespoons pastured lard or other healthy fat of choice
½ head Napa cabbage or other cabbage of choice, shredded (about 4 cups)
2 large carrots, cut into matchsticks

2 bell peppers, any color, cut into matchsticks
4 radishes, sliced
1 bunch green onions, thinly sliced
1 cup pistachios or macadamia nuts, chopped
1 cup chopped cilantro leaves (optional)
½ cup chopped regular or Thai basil
Fresh black pepper

Dressing
Makes 2 cups (leftovers can be stored in the fridge)

¾ cup coconut vinegar or apple cider vinegar
1 cup cold-pressed sesame oil
¼ cup coconut aminos
Juice of 1 lime
2 tablespoons minced garlic
¼ cup fresh ginger, shredded with a microplane zester or finely chopped
1 jalapeño pepper, seeded and finely chopped (optional; for added spice, leave the seeds in)
Sea salt and pepper

Preheat the oven 350°F. Generously salt and pepper the chicken on both sides. Add the fat to a cast-iron skillet and heat to medium-high. Pan-sear the chicken for about 3 to 5 minutes per side, then place in the oven for an additional 15 minutes.

While chicken is cooking, assemble your salad. Toss together in a large bowl the cabbage, carrots, peppers, radishes, and onions. In a smaller bowl, whisk the dressing ingredients. Take the chicken out of the oven, and let it rest for 5 minutes before slicing it into strips and placing them on top of the salad. Pour the dressing over the top, reserving some for the table (or your fridge). Sprinkle with the chopped nuts, fresh herbs, and a generous crack of pepper. Beautiful!

FENNEL AND LEMON SALAD
Serves 4 to 6

This is delicious and refreshing, and it's surprisingly kid-friendly, too. It's a great side salad, and not a protein/lunch salad. I love serving it alongside any simple fish dish.

3 fennel bulbs, sliced thinly or diced
Juice and zest of 1 lemon
½ head fresh parsley, chopped
Fennel fronds, as a garnish
Sea salt and pepper
2 tablespoons olive oil

Chop off the long stalks of the fennel, cut the bulb in half, and remove the outermost layer. Save some of the wispy fennel fronds to add to the salad. Slice the fennel bulb, then chop it into ½-inch pieces. Add the lemon juice and zest, parsley, and fennel fronds, then salt and pepper to taste. Drizzle with two big glugs of olive oil, toss, and serve.

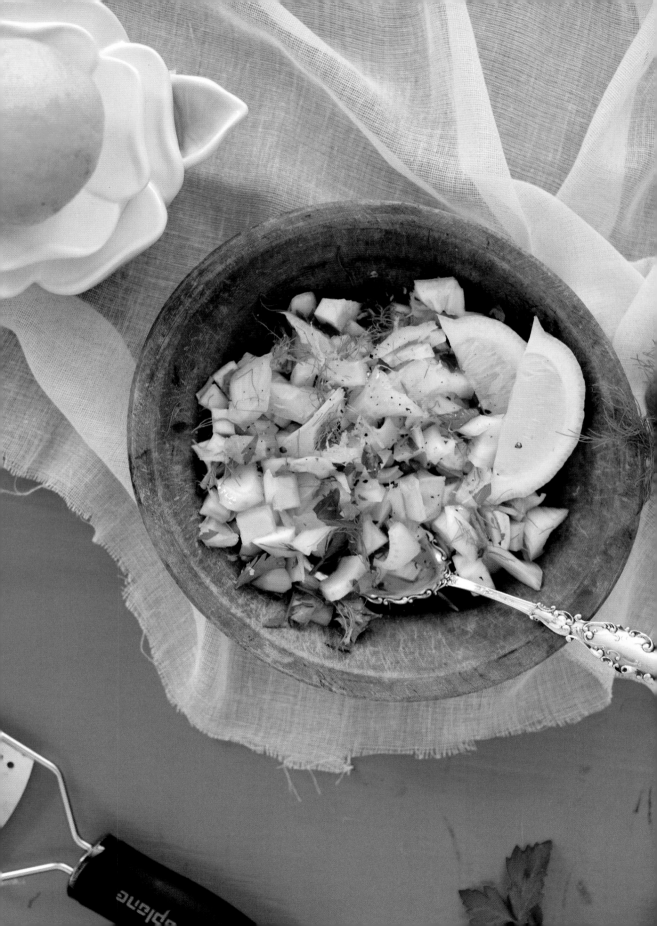

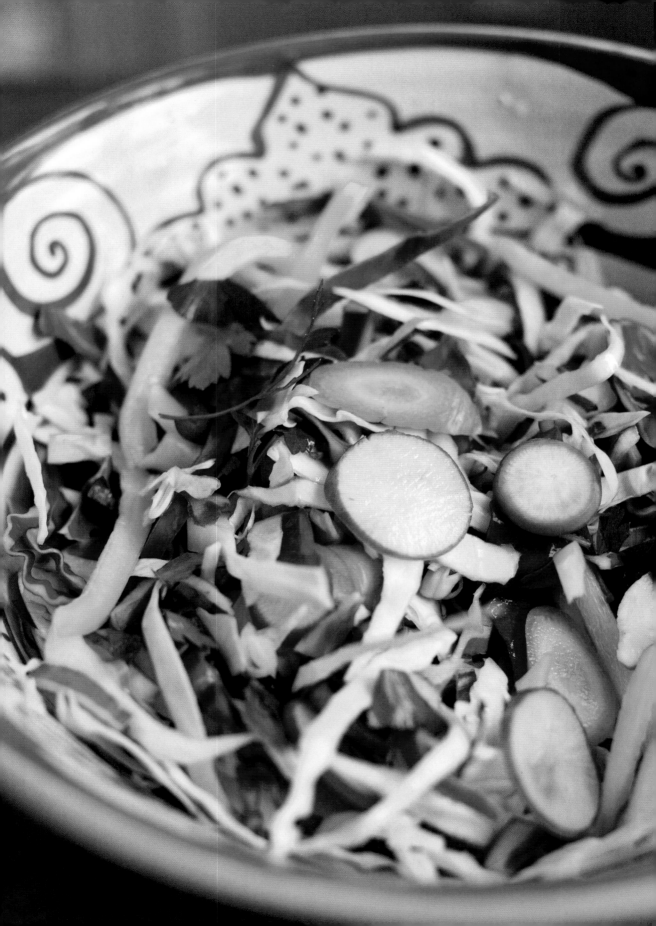

CABBAGE SALAD TWO WAYS

Raw cabbage should be eaten only occasionally, as it can have thyroid-suppressing effects when consumed in large amounts. If you have trouble digesting this, back off and wait until your gut issues have had a bit longer to heal or substitute a head of Romaine lettuce or greens of your choice for the cabbage. This is inspired by good old Jamie Oliver . . . love him!

Basic Recipe
Serves 6 to 8

½ white cabbage, shredded
½ red cabbage, shredded
Good pinch of salt
½ red onion, sliced
4 sliced radishes

1 bunch cilantro or parsley
1 carrot, sliced in rounds
1 jalapeño, seeded and chopped
   (optional)
2–3 scallions, for garnish

DRESSING
Makes ½ cup

3–4 tablespoons olive oil
1 tablespoon coconut vinegar or apple
   cider vinegar
1 tablespoon honey (optional)

Juice and zest of 1 lime
¼ cup 24-hour cultured yogurt or
   kefir (optional)
Sea salt and pepper

Red Cabbage and Mango (beautiful with salmon)
Serves 6 to 8

1 red cabbage
Good pinch of salt

1 mango, diced
1 bunch cilantro

DRESSING

2 tablespoons coconut vinegar
3–4 tablespoons olive oil
Juice and zest of 1 lime
1 tablespoon honey (optional)
Sea salt and pepper

Shred the cabbage, add the salt, and massage for about a minute to soften and break down the cellulose. Add the remaining ingredients, toss with the dressing, and season to taste.

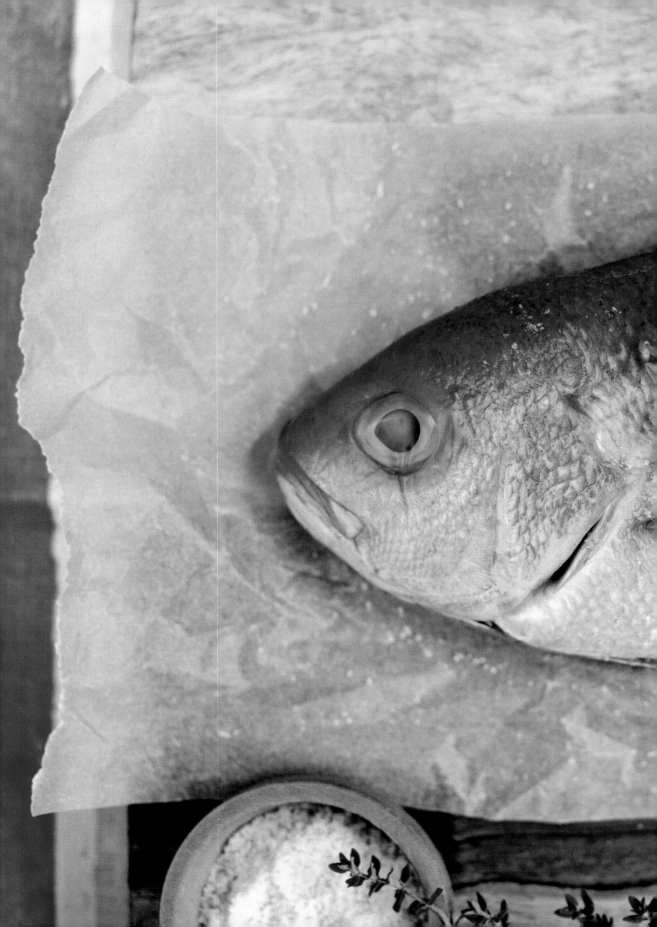

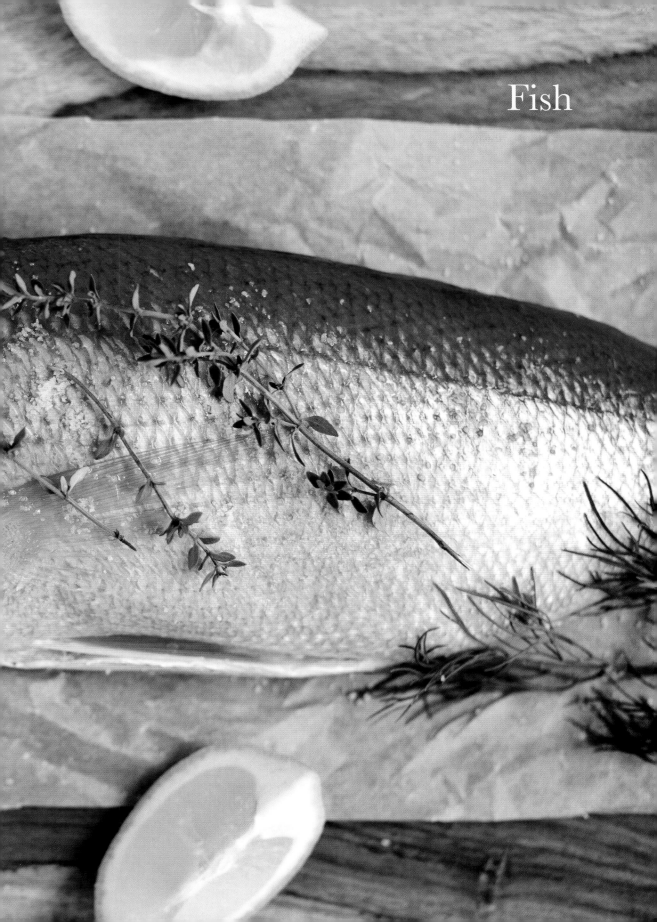

Fish

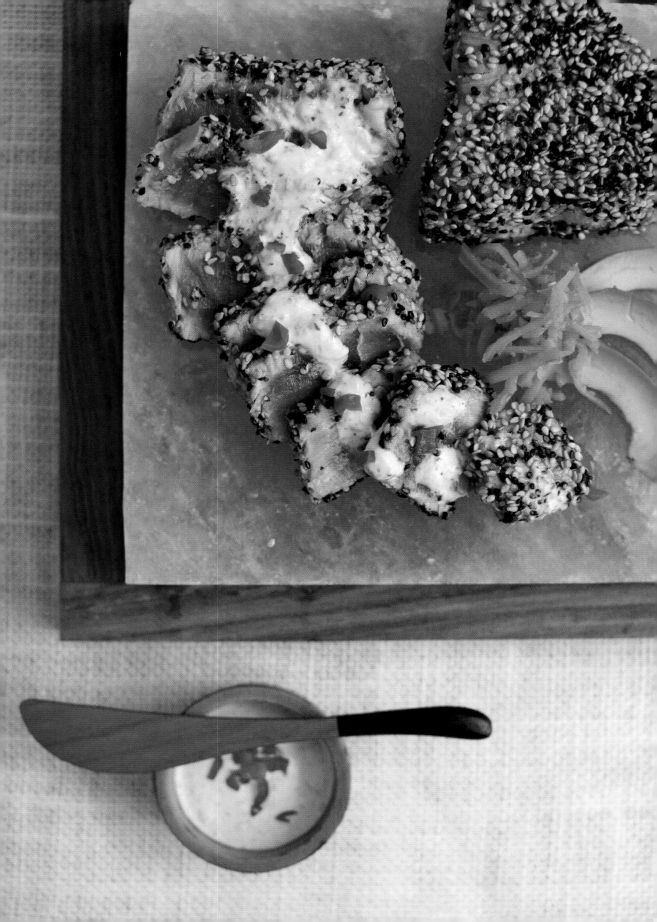

BLACK SESAME SEARED TUNA SASHIMI
Serves 2 to 4

Four of my five kids love tuna sashimi, which has saved us more than once when choosing from a restaurant menu. I've created my own to make at home, and it has become a favorite appetizer, dinner, and even school lunch (packed on ice). I use my homemade mayo blended with Hot Nicky for a kick, but you could certainly mix wasabi powder and filtered water, too, as long as it has no fillers or suspicious ingredients.

¼ cup black sesame seeds
¼ cup white sesame seeds
1 teaspoon sea salt
Freshly ground black pepper
2 tuna steaks, sushi-grade
   (about 1½ pounds)
2 tablespoons ghee or coconut oil
Salad greens
2 ripe avocados, sliced thin
Fermented Ginger Carrots (page 235)
Hot Nicky (page 241) mixed with
   homemade mayonnaise (page 107)

Combine the sesame seeds, salt, and pepper in a bowl. Coat the tuna on all sides, pressing the mixture onto the fish so the seeds will stick. Heat the ghee or coconut oil in a skillet. Be sure to get the pan nice and hot. Cook the steaks one at a time without crowding the pan (to ensure even cooking), about 1 minute on each side. Then, using tongs, sear the edges for about 20 seconds each. This will make for a nice rare steak. Serve alongside or on top of fresh salad greens and top with avocado, Ginger Carrots (page 235), and a dap of cultured cream or Hot Nicky Mayo.

SALMON WITH HOMEMADE GARLIC AIOLI
Serves 4 to 8

This is one of our family's favorite "fast-food" meals, perfect for when time is tight. I always try to keep some wild salmon in the freezer; it will thaw out in 5 to 10 minutes! One of the boys, along with our cat, loves the skin, so he collects it from everyone's plate. It thrills me that he's getting such great fats into his diet! If aioli isn't an option, try this dish with Pesto (page 114) or Guacamole (page 116)

1–2 pounds salmon fillet
2–3 tablespoons coconut oil
Sea salt and pepper
Lemon juice
Handful of fresh parsley (optional)

Preheat the oven to 350°F. Place the salmon in a pan, and add a few dollops of coconut oil on top. Sprinkle with salt and pepper and a squeeze of fresh lemon juice. Slip into the oven, and bake for 15 minutes. Garnish with fresh chopped parsley, and serve alongside Garlic Aioli (page 108).

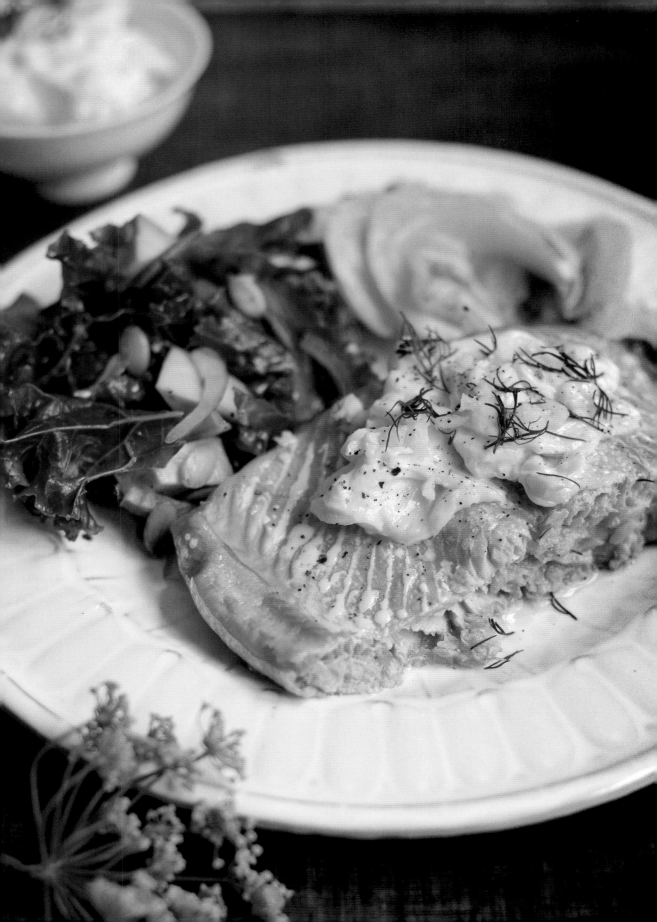

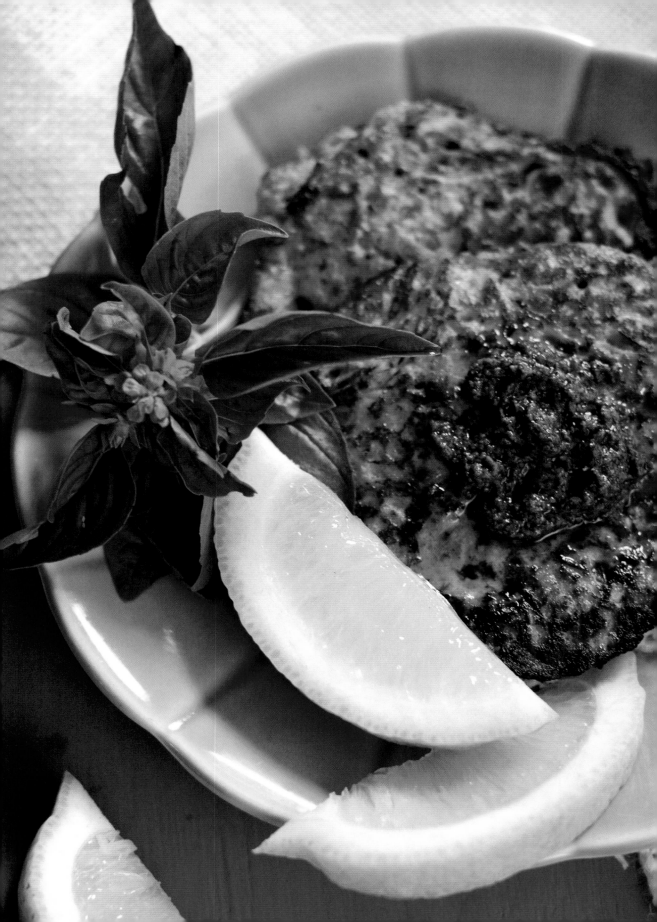

SALMON CAKES WITH LEMON PESTO
Serves 4

1 5–6 oz can boneless, skinless wild
  Alaskan salmon, *or* 1 cup cooked wild
  salmon, flaked with a fork
⅓ cup squash puree (page 70)
3 pastured eggs
Sea salt and black pepper
2 tablespoons minced red or white onion
½ bunch fresh parsley, chopped
Fat for the pan, such as ghee or
  coconut oil

Mix the salmon and squash together with a fork. Stir in the eggs, salt, pepper, onion, and parsley. Make into patties about ¾ inch thick.

Heat 2 tablespoons of fat in a skillet. Cook the Salmon Cakes in batches, 2 to 3 minutes per side. Add fat as needed for each new batch. Serve on a bed of fresh greens with Lemon Pesto (recipe follows).

Lemon Pesto
Makes approximately 1 pint

2–3 garlic cloves
¼ cup toasted pine nuts or
  walnuts (a less expensive option)
2 cups loosely packed fresh basil leaves
½ cup loosely packed fresh flat-leaf
  parsley leaves
¼ cup grated raw Parmigiano-Reggiano
  (optional)
1 teaspoon lemon zest
1 tablespoon fresh lemon juice
1–1½ cups extra-virgin olive oil
Sea salt and freshly ground pepper

Combine all of the ingredients in a food processor or Vitamix and blend well. While the machine is running, slowly drizzle in the olive oil until you reach your desired consistency. Season with salt and pepper. Put in a pint-sized mason jar, and store in the fridge.

ZUCCHINI FRITTERS
Serves 4

1 medium zucchini, grated
2 pastured eggs
1 clove garlic, minced
Sea salt and pepper
3 tablespoons coconut oil, ghee, or
   preferred fat for frying

Mix all of the ingredients (except the fat) together, and follow Salmon Cakes' cooking instructions (page 151). Serve with Cultured Cream and Kefir Herb Dressing (page 127).

MARINATED CODFISH TACOS WITH COCONUT FLOUR TORTILLAS
Serves 6 to 8

This dish uses a marinade that would work with any light fish, from haddock to sole to cod; it would even be great on salmon. If you are unable to handle coconut flour due to digestive issues, please substitute Cumin Cauliflower Crepes (page 86) for the tortillas.

½ fennel bulb
1 red onion
2 cloves garlic
1 teaspoon sea salt
½ teaspoon fresh cracked black pepper
Zest of 2 limes
1–2 teaspoons cumin
1 jalapeño or other hot chile, seeded or not . . . (optional)
1½ cups olive oil
½ bunch cilantro (or herb of choice) plus ½ bunch cilantro, for garnish
2–4 pounds cod, or fish of choice
Juice of 1 lime

Roughly chop the fennel bulb and red onion and place in your food processor. Add the garlic, salt and pepper, lime zest, cumin, and jalapeño or chile, and pulse until everything is finely chopped. Add the olive oil and cilantro, and pulse to incorporate. Pour into a glass container. This marinade will stay fresh in the fridge for 1 week; it's enough for two or three dinners.

Cut the fish into 2-inch chunks, and place them in a glass dish. Cover with the marinade, seal, and leave in the fridge for at least 2 hours, preferably overnight.

Grill the fish on skewers (it's very pretty alternating with yellow zucchini and red onion). Or you may also pour the fish and marinade into a glass dish and bake at 350°F for 15 to 17 minutes.

Squeeze fresh lime juice and sprinkle chopped cilantro over the fish and serve as is, or wrap it in coconut flour tortillas (recipe follows) with lettuce, guacamole, cultured cream, and fermented salsa or fresh chopped tomatoes.

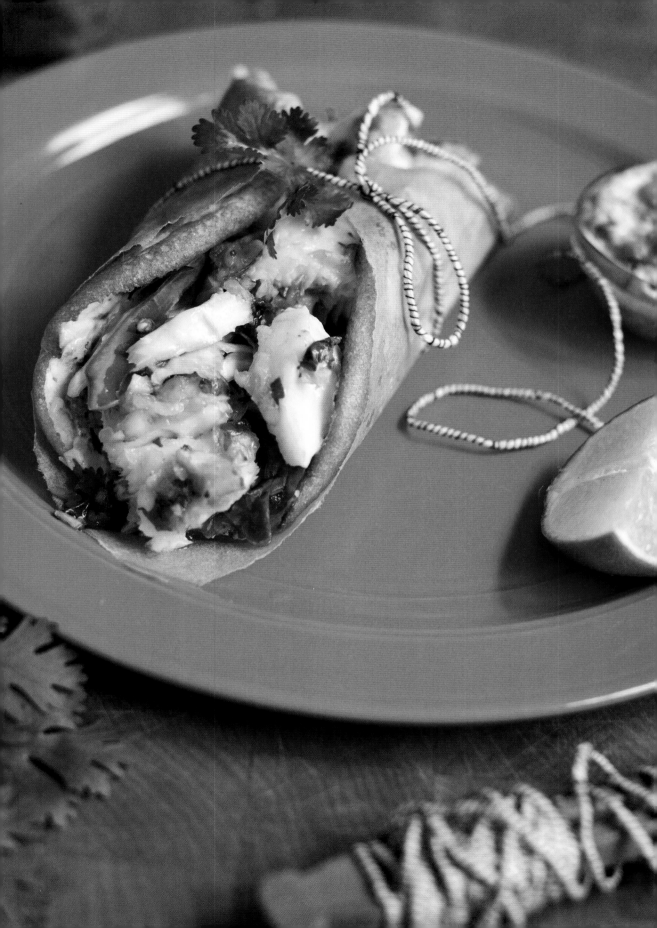

Coconut Flour Tortillas
Makes 4 tortillas

6 egg whites plus 2 whole eggs
½ cup coconut milk (or ½ cup filtered
    water) (page 23)
¼ cup coconut flour (page 26)

¼ teaspoon sea salt
¼ teaspoon lemon juice
Coconut oil or lard for cooking

FOR MEXICAN TORTILLA, ADD:

½ teaspoon garlic powder
½ teaspoon cumin
½ teaspoon onion powder

Combine all of the ingredients (except the fat) in a food processor or whisk together in a bowl, making sure to break up all the lumps in the batter. Heat 1 tablespoon of the coconut oil in a nonstick pan, and pour in 3 to 4 tablespoons batter. Move the pan around to evenly distribute a thin layer of batter in a round tortilla shape. Cook on medium heat until the tortilla is nicely browned on one side, about 1½ minutes. Work around the edges with a rubber spatula, and carefully flip the tortilla and cook on the other side for an additional minute. Slide out onto a plate and repeat. Make sure to add coconut oil to the pan in between tortillas. Store in a sealed container in the fridge for a few days. Be sure to use the leftover egg yolks to make the Lemon Curd (page 95), Homemade Mayo (pages 107–108), or toss in your Power Smoothie (page 96).

SALT-AND-PEPPER SHRIMP
Serves 6 to 8

4–5 tablespoons coconut oil
4 cloves garlic, pressed
2 pounds wild shrimp, peeled and deveined
2 tablespoons fresh lemon juice
½ teaspoon sea salt
1 teaspoon black pepper
2 tablespoons chopped parsley

In a sauté pan over medium heat, warm the coconut oil. Add the garlic; sauté for 1 minute, until fragrant. Increase the heat to high, add the shrimp and lemon juice, stir well, and sauté until the shrimp turn pink and are opaque throughout, about 3 minutes. Season with salt and black pepper, sprinkle with parsley, and serve with your sauce of choice (recipes follow).

Garlic and Chive Aioli

¼ cup mayo
1 clove garlic, chopped
Handful of fresh chives, chopped

Mix all of the ingredients together in a small bowl; drizzle over the shrimp or serve on the side.

Hot Nicky Aioli

¼ cup mayo (page 107)
1 clove garlic, chopped
1 tablespoon Hot Nicky (page 241)

Mix all of the ingredients together in a small bowl; drizzle over the shrimp or serve on the side.

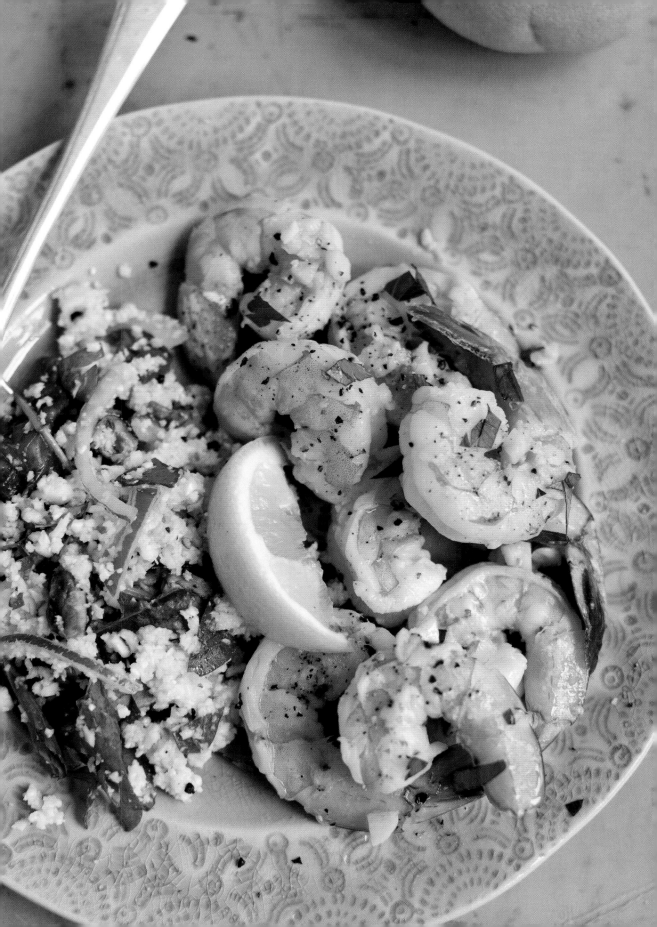

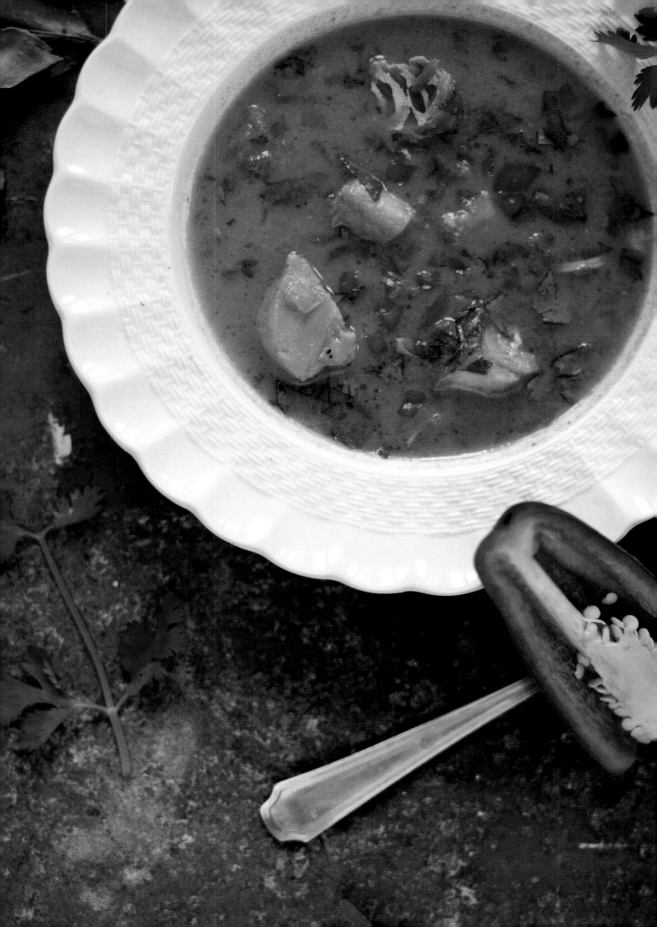

COCONUT CURRY FISH STEW
Serves 8 to 10

I used to be intimidated by recipes with more than a few ingredients. But I promise that this is an easy one. If you don't have the lemongrass or kaffir lime leaves, just add a little fresh lemon and lime zest . . . don't sweat it either way. This is well worth it, and once you make it, you'll see how easy it is to throw together.

2 tablespoons coconut oil

2 onions, diced

3 inches fresh gingerroot, minced

2–4 jalapeño peppers, seeds and ribs removed, minced

3 garlic cloves, minced

3 tablespoons curry powder

¼ teaspoon turmeric

⅛ teaspoon cayenne

1 tablespoon sea salt

½ teaspoon fresh ground black pepper

2 quarts (8 cups) chicken or fish broth or stock (you can use half filtered water, half stock if you desire)

1 can full-fat coconut milk (homemade, page 23, or Native Forest brand without guar gum)

1 can (28 ounces) organic crushed tomatoes

1 red bell pepper, diced

3 sticks dried lemongrass

3 kaffir lime leaves

2 pounds cod or haddock, cut into 2-inch cubes

½ cup chopped fresh cilantro, plus more for garnish

Lime zest, for garnish

Avocado, diced

Heat the oil in a saucepan. Add the onions, and sauté for a good 5 minutes, until soft. Add the ginger, jalapeño, and garlic, and sauté for another few minutes. Add the spices, and toss with the onion mixture, stirring for about 2 minutes. Add the stock, coconut milk, tomatoes, bell pepper, lemongrass, and kaffir lime leaves; bring to a boil. Reduce the heat to a simmer for 25 minutes. Add the fish and cilantro, and cook for an additional 10 minutes. Garnish with lime zest, diced avocado, and more cilantro, and serve.

Variation: To switch things up a bit, try using diced chicken instead of fish.

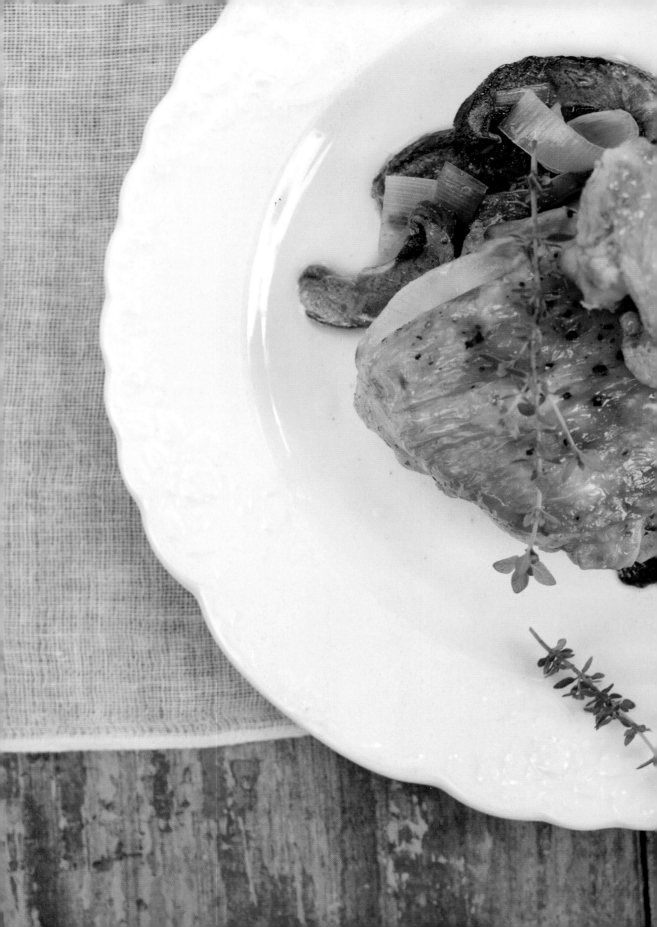

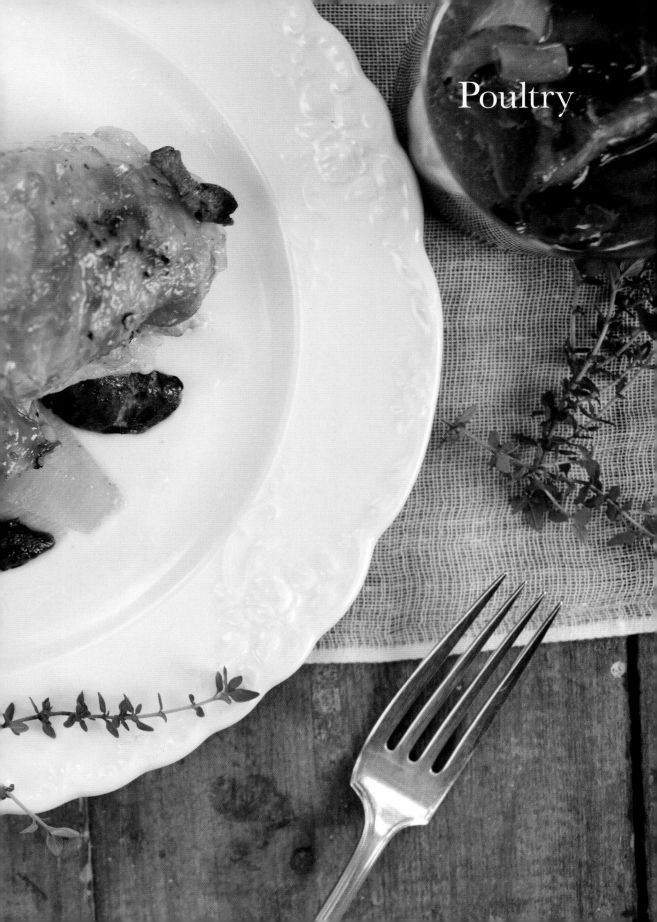

Poultry

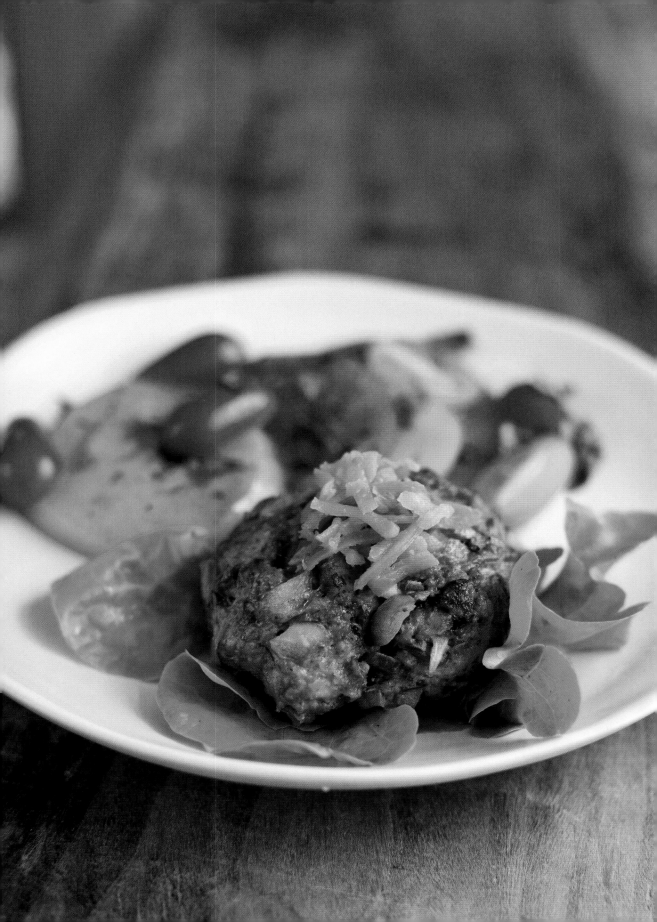

CILANTRO TURKEY BURGERS
Makes 8 burgers

These are delicious with guacamole, salsa, and chipotle mayo. Even though we eat our burgers without bread, the Coconut Butter Bread works great as a bun replacement if you are looking for something to hold it all together!

2 pounds ground turkey
2 cloves garlic, minced
½ bunch cilantro
1 red onion, chopped
1 tablespoon chili powder
1 teaspoon sea salt
Fresh cracked pepper
3 slices Coconut Butter Bread (page 118),
    torn into chunks (optional)
½ cup homemade sour cream (optional)

Turn your oven to broil. Place all of the ingredients (except the bread and sour cream) in a bowl and gently mix together with your hands. If you have kids who may not like chunks of onion in their burger, you can leave the onion out, or grate or blend it in your food processor until finely chopped. Form the mixture into burger patties. Broil in your oven for 5 to 7 minutes per side (check to be sure they are cooked throughout). If you have any digestive issues, or are not eating dairy, just leave out the Coconut Butter Bread and the sour cream. They will still be just as delicious. You can also individually wrap these in parchment paper and then foil, and freeze. This is a great option if you are eating alone or need to pack something for overnight at a friend's house.

MARINATED CHICKEN WINGS
Makes 25 to 30 wings

A couple of years ago, I served on the board of a great nonprofit called Gaining Ground, which grows tons of organic vegetables to feed people in need. Their head farmer, Verena, who knows a thing or two about preserving the harvest's bounty, told me that I could freeze my jalapeños. What a great tip! If you have ever grown jalapeño plants, you know that they produce a lot. Personally, I don't go through a hundred jalapeños in a summer. So now I have a nice big bag in my freezer, and I pull them out as needed. If you want to preserve the most flavor, roast them at 400°F for 15 minutes before freezing.

¼ cup honey (optional)
2 tablespoons apple cider vinegar
¼ cup coconut aminos
1 onion, finely chopped
1 tablespoon ghee, schmaltz (chicken fat), lard, or butter, melted
1 red chile or jalapeño, diced (remove seeds, optional)
1–2 inches gingerroot, grated
2 cloves garlic, minced
Pinch of cayenne (optional)
25–30 chicken wings and/or drumsticks
½ teaspoon sea salt
2 tablespoons sesame seeds
Chopped scallions, for garnish

In a medium saucepan over medium-low heat, gently melt together the honey, apple cider vinegar, and coconut aminos until incorporated. Add the remaining ingredients (except the chicken, salt, sesame seeds, and scallions) and stir. Place the chicken in a giant glass or porcelain baking dish. Pour the marinade over it, making sure all the wings are covered. Massage the marinade into the wings, cover, and place in the fridge for at least 2 hours (preferably overnight, tossing two or three times).

Preheat the oven to 425°F. Spread the chicken wings on a large pan and sprinkle with salt. Bake for 25 to 30 minutes, until cooked through and nicely browned on the top. Sprinkle with sesame seeds and chopped scallions and serve. If you are worried about spices, you can omit the chile and cayenne.

Note: *In a pinch I have popped the wings on a sheet pan, drizzled them with coconut aminos, chopped garlic, and ginger, added a few pinches of salt and pepper, tossed, and then popped them in the oven. Upon removing, I sprinkle with sesame seeds and serve! If you don't have time for marinating, don't sweat it!*

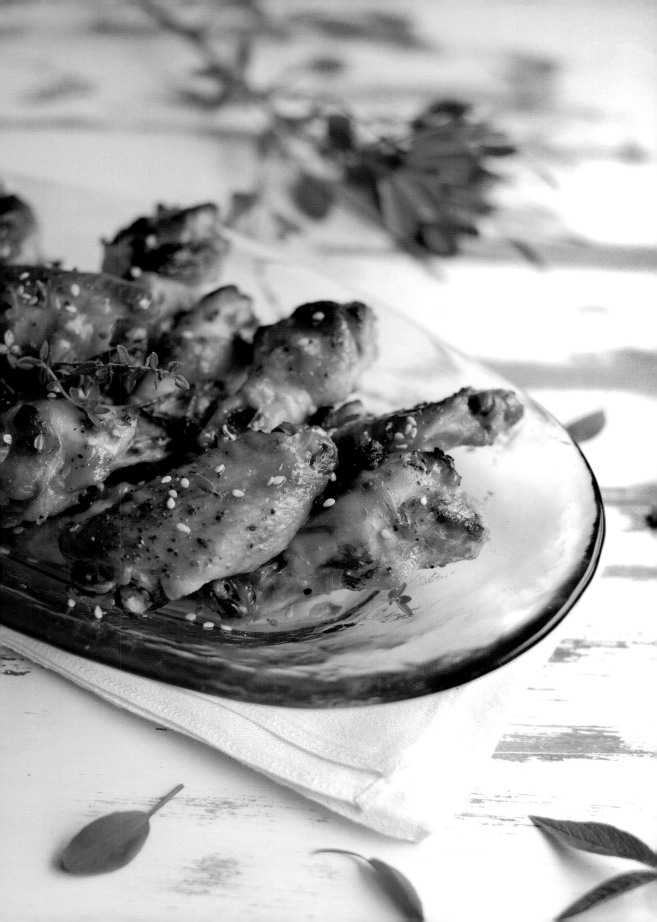

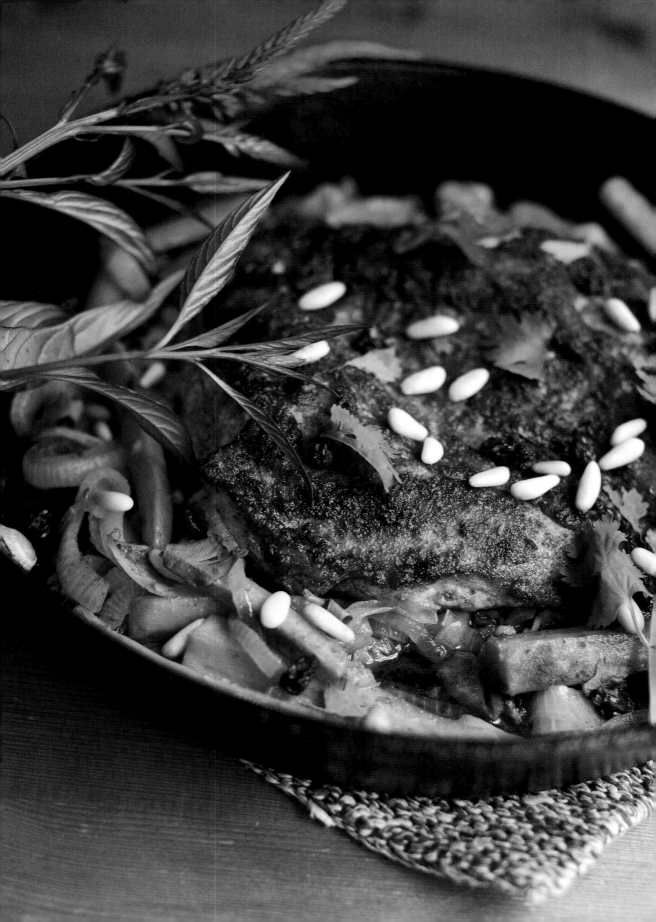

MOROCCAN CHICKEN
Serves 4 to 6

The diced preserved lemons make this delicious dish taste really authentic! You can add this spice mix to any vegetables; cauliflower is particularly great. To do so, simply coat with palm or coconut oil, toss with spices, and roast for 50 minutes at 350°F.

3–4 carrots, cut into sticks

2 onions, sliced in rings

3 tablespoons palm oil (I like it best with palm oil, but feel free to use a healthy fat of your choice), divided

3 cloves garlic, chopped

1–2 inches fresh gingerroot, peeled and chopped

1 teaspoon sea salt

1½ teaspoons paprika

1 teaspoon turmeric

2 teaspoons cumin

1 teaspoon coriander

Fresh cracked pepper

1–2 pounds skin-on chicken parts: breasts, thighs, and/or legs

1 cup chicken broth or stock

¼ cup raisins

¼ cup pine nuts, lightly toasted

½ bunch fresh cilantro or parsley, chopped

Preserved lemon, diced (recipe follows; optional)

Preheat the oven to 350°F. In a large ovenproof skillet over medium heat, sauté the carrots and onions in half the palm oil for 10 minutes. Add the garlic and ginger; sauté for another 5 to 10 minutes. While the carrots and onions are sautéing, mix your spices in a little bowl. Coat the chicken in spices. Heat the second half of the palm oil in another pan and add the chicken, skin-side down. Let it cook for 3 to 4 minutes, flip, and cook for an additional 3 to 4 minutes. Place the chicken on top of the carrots and onions, add the chicken stock, then put the skillet in the oven for 15 to 20 minutes. Slice the chicken, and garnish with raisins, pine nuts, herbs, and chopped preserved lemon (page 168); season with additional salt and pepper, if needed.

Preserved Lemons
Makes 1 to 2 pints

This is an easy great recipe inspired by my friend Alex Lewin, author of *Real Food Fermentation.*

1½ pounds organic lemons and/or limes, at room temperature
¼ cup sea salt
Assorted spices of choice: a cinnamon stick, a bay leaf, a few cloves, a few peppercorns, a handful of coriander seeds, or a shake of pickling spice
1 pint-sized mason jar with tight-fitting lid

Wash the lemons or limes. Cut each piece of fruit in half, then score deeply with an X across the inside of each half. Discard the seeds. Put some salt in the bottom of the jar, then add some spices and a fruit's worth of wedges (cut-side down). Repeat layer by layer until the jar is full, leaving 1 inch at top. Press down firmly to make sure all of the fruit is covered by juices. If you need to top off the jar, use the juice from one more fruit. Close the jar, and store at room temperature out of direct sunlight. Leave on the counter for a week, opening daily to pack down the fruit. Leave out, as flavor will deepen throughout the year—or you can place the jar in the fridge at any time to slow down the fermentation.

SHREDDED TACO CHICKEN IN A CROCK-POT
Serves 6 to 8

I *love* Kelly the Kitchen Kop for giving me this quick option. It is absolutely the way to go when you are in a rush and have to schlep kids to soccer practice or events all afternoon and have zero time to cook. All you have to do when you get home is whip up some guacamole, chop some tomatoes, pull out some lettuce and the ferments . . . and you have a delicious shredded chicken taco salad. Feel free to substitute grass-fed beef cubes or rump roast for the chicken, too!

2 cups chicken broth, stock, or filtered water
2 tablespoons lard, ghee, or fat of choice
¼ cup Taco Seasoning (page 128)
2 pounds boneless chicken breasts (this is the best tip: You can throw them into the Crock-Pot frozen solid!

In the morning, put all of the ingredients into your Crock-Pot on low. Let it cook all day on low (5 to 6 hours), and when the chicken falls apart easily, use a fork to shred it right in the Crock-Pot. Enjoy the delicious cooking juices, too! If you have a VitaClay (see resources), this can be cooked in 1 to 2 hours!

STACKED CHICKEN SANDWICH
Serves 4

You might want to use a knife and fork . . .

1 whole skin-on chicken breast
Sea salt and pepper
2 tablespoons coconut oil or animal fat

Preheat the oven to 350°F. Season both sides of chicken with salt and pepper. In an ovenproof skillet, melt the fat over medium-high heat. Pan-sear the chicken, skin-side down, for 3 to 4 minutes, then flip and cook for an additional 3 to 4 minutes. Place in the oven for 15 to 20 minutes. Remove, let cool, and slice.

Add-ons for one serving:

- 2 slices Coconut Butter Bread, toasted (page 118)
- 2 tablespoons homemade mayonnaise (page 107)
- ¼ sliced avocado
- 1 small handful of fresh greens or sprouts
- Homemade Red Cabbage, Raisin, and Apple Sauerkraut (page 236)
- Sliced raw cheddar cheese (optional)
- Fermented pickle slices (I love the brands Bubbies and Real Pickles)
- Lacto-Fermented Mustard (page 109)

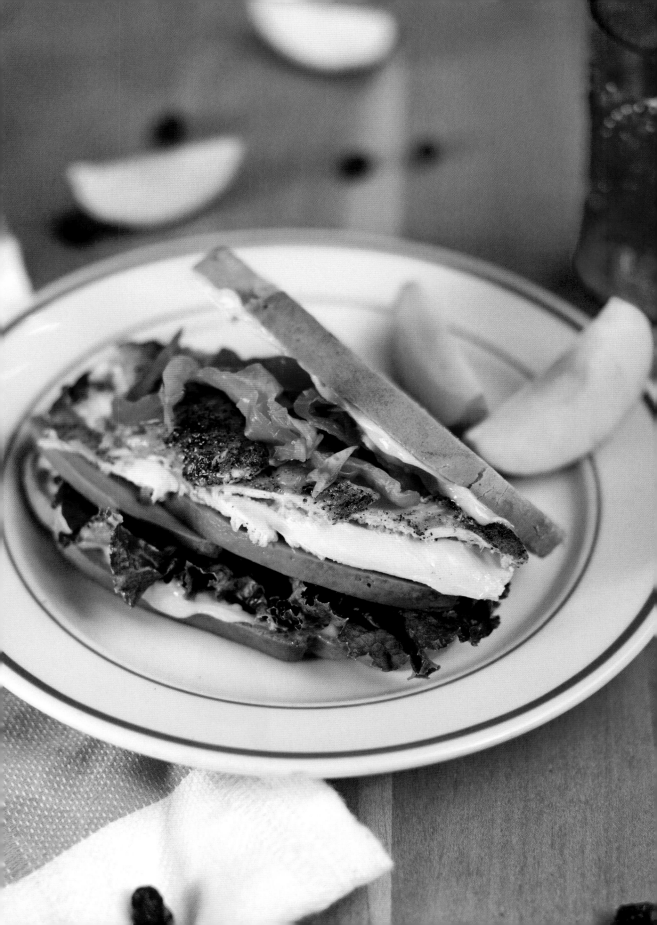

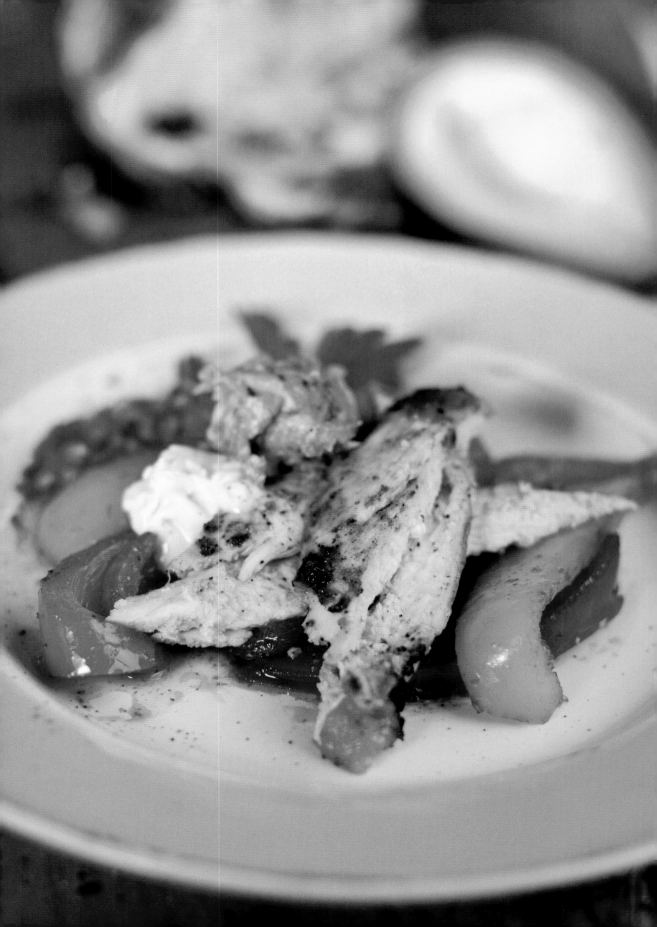

MEXICAN CHICKEN WITH LACTO-FERMENTED SALSA
Serves 4 to 6

This is very popular in our house!

2 tablespoons coconut oil, lard, or
    preferred fat, divided
3 white onions, sliced in rings
Sea salt and pepper
2 bell peppers, any color, sliced
2–3 tablespoons Taco Seasoning
    (page 128)
Juice and zest of 2 limes
1 whole chicken breast, skin on, or 8
    skin-on chicken thighs (chicken thighs
    are higher in fat, so these may be more
    desirable than the breast)
1–2 tablespoons olive oil
Handful of fresh cilantro, chopped,
    for garnish

Preheat the oven to 350°F. In a large saucepan, heat 1 tablespoon of fat and add the onions. Add a pinch of salt, and sauté for about 5 minutes before adding the peppers. Throw in a tablespoon of the Taco Seasoning and a squeeze of fresh lime juice, and continue to sauté for 30 to 45 minutes to caramelize the onions and peppers.

Heat the remaining 1 tablespoon of fat in an ovenproof skillet. Salt and pepper the chicken on both sides, then season with the remaining Taco Seasoning, making sure to coat the entire breast. Place the chicken, skin-side down, in the hot pan. Cook for 4 to 5 minutes, turn over, and cook for an additional 3 to 4 minutes on the other side. Place in the oven for 15 minutes, remove, and let rest for 5 minutes. Slice the chicken in strips and serve alongside the peppers and onions. Zest 1 lime and squeeze its juice over the entire dish. Drizzle with olive oil and sprinkle with chopped cilantro to garnish. Serve with home-made guacamole (page 116), cultured cream (page 30), chopped cilantro, and Lacto-Fermented Cilantro Salsa (page 234).

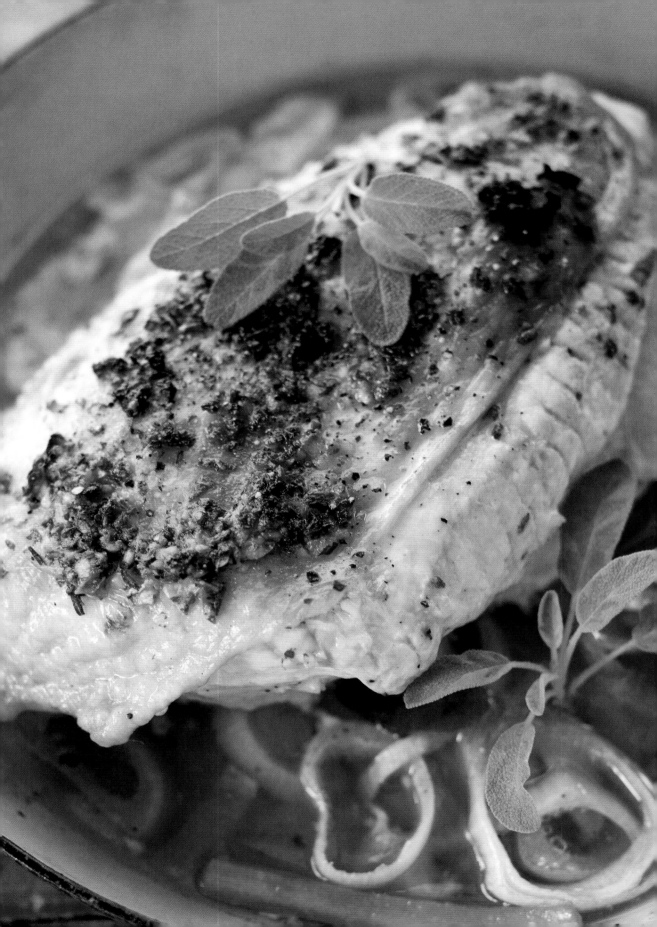

HERB-ROASTED TURKEY BREAST
Serves 8 to 10

I can't believe I ever actually purchased those overpriced organic turkey breast cold cuts for $1 a slice. Roasting a turkey breast is even easier than roasting a chicken! It's a huge money saver, and as a bonus it also makes a delicious broth. The amazing Ina Garten helped me out with this one; I have adapted her recipe a bit for GAPS.

3 carrots, roughly chopped

2 onions, sliced

4 cloves garlic, 2 minced for paste and 2 smashed for broth

Additional vegetables, such as fennel, leeks, or celery, roughly chopped (optional)

2–3 cups chicken broth or stock

1 teaspoon sea salt, plus a couple pinches

1 teaspoon fresh ground pepper, plus a couple pinches

1 3-pound turkey breast (double all other ingredients for a 6-pound breast)

1 tablespoon dried sage

1 tablespoon dried thyme

1 tablespoon dried rosemary

1 teaspoon dry mustard

Juice of ½ lemon

2 tablespoons lard, coconut oil, ghee, or butter

1–2 tablespoons gelatin

Preheat the oven to 325°F. Place the carrots, onions, smashed garlic cloves, vegetables, and broth in the bottom of your Dutch oven or roasting pan. Season with pinches of salt and pepper. Place the breast, skin-side up, on top of the vegetables.

In a small bowl, combine the spices, minced garlic, lemon juice, 1 teaspoon salt, 1 teaspoon pepper, and fat of your choice. Mash into a paste. Lift the skin of the breast and smear half of the paste underneath. Rub the remaining paste over the rest of the breast.

Place the roasting pan in the preheated oven for 50 minutes to 1 hour. Baste the turkey halfway through the cooking time with the broth and pan juices. Remove from the oven when a thermometer inserted in the thickest part of the breast reads 165°F. Tent the turkey with foil, and allow it to rest for 15 minutes before carving.

You can strain off the broth and drink it as is (delicious), or you can make a fabulous gravy with those juices. Remove the vegetables to a serving plate, then put the pan on the stovetop over medium heat (you may wish to remove some broth, which will make for a thicker gravy). Whisk in the gelatin by the tablespoon until you have thickened the juices a bit. It might not be a super-thick gravy, but it is still yummy. Add salt and pepper to taste, and pour over the turkey breast.

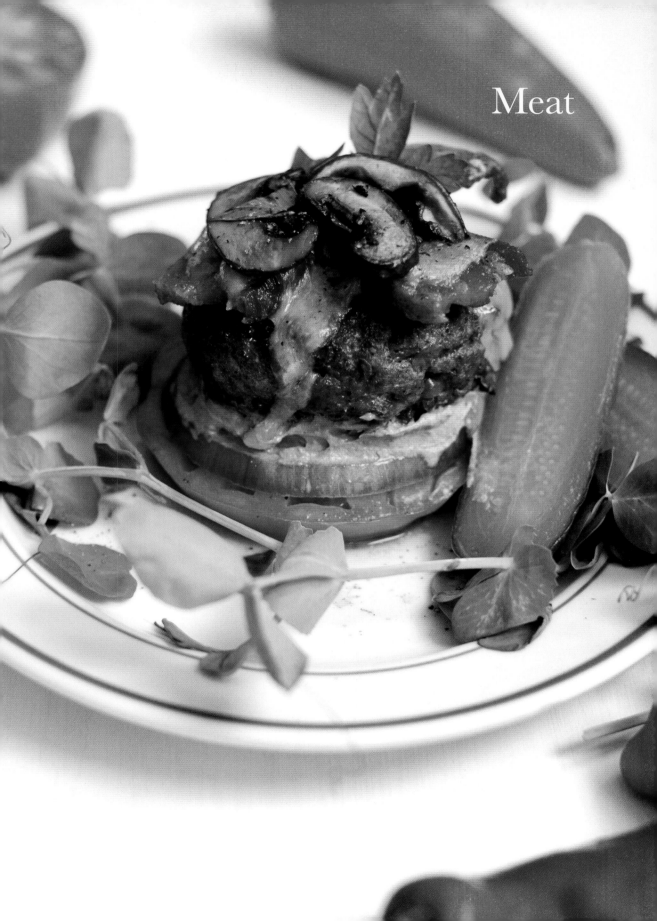

Meat

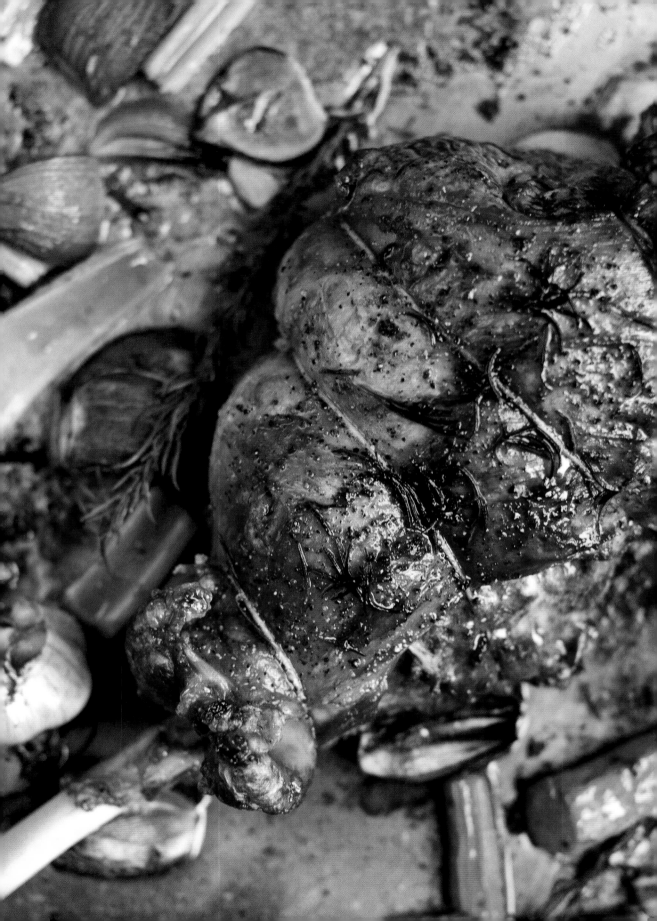

LEG OF LAMB TWO WAYS

Oven-Roasted Leg of Lamb with Mint Sauce and Kefir Cheese
Serves 8 to 10

Leg of lamb is a big Easter tradition in my family. I remember eating it with bright green mint jelly (who knows what that was) while the grown-ups enjoyed the more traditional mint sauce. I have opted to give you the latter, GAPS-style!

1 4-pound leg of lamb

4 red onions, quartered

4 carrots, roughly chopped

4 celery stalks, roughly chopped

¼ cup chopped fresh herbs of choice
   (I like rosemary and thyme)

1 bay leaf

¼ cup animal fat of choice, warmed: lard,
   lamb, or beef tallow

5 cloves garlic, slightly crushed with
   side of knife

Sea salt and pepper

Take the lamb out of the fridge, and allow it to come to room temperature (about 30 minutes). Preheat your oven to 475°F. Place the vegetables and fresh herbs, along with the bay leaf, in the bottom of a roasting pan; drizzle with the fat. Place the lamb on top of the vegetables. Make five slits in meat, and slide a whole garlic clove in each. Generously season the entire pan with salt and fresh cracked pepper.

Place in the oven, and turn it down to 450°F. Cook the lamb for 20 minutes. At this point, baste the lamb and check the vegetables to make sure they aren't burning. If they're too dry, add some filtered water or stock to the pan. Reduce the heat again to 325°F, and cook for another 40 minutes. A meat thermometer inserted into the thickest part of the leg should read 145 to 150°F. This will be perfectly pink in the middle. Remove the lamb, tent it with foil, and let it rest for an additional 30 minutes. Carve the lamb with a sharp carving knife. Serve with Mint Sauce and Rosemary Kefir Cheese (recipes follow).

MINT SAUCE
Serves 8 to 10

⅓ cup raw honey
1 large bunch fresh mint, minced
¼ cup coconut vinegar
Sea salt and pepper

Whisk the honey with the remaining ingredients. Add a little hot filtered water if needed to thin out the consistency. Serve in a bowl with a spoon alongside the lamb. Store in the fridge.

ROSEMARY KEFIR CHEESE
Makes approximately 1 cup

Follow the yogurt cheese instructions (page 32) using 1 quart raw kefir or yogurt. Combine with:

2 cloves garlic, pressed
1 tablespoon chopped fresh
  rosemary or thyme

Sea salt and pepper
Big drizzle of olive oil

"Slow and Low" Roasted Leg of Lamb with Gravy
Serves 8 to 10

1 4-pound leg of lamb
¼ cup animal fat of choice, warmed: lard,
  lamb, or beef tallow
4 red onions, quartered
4 carrots, roughly chopped
4 celery stalks, roughly chopped
2 cups broth or stock
1 bottle dry red wine
¼ cup chopped fresh herbs of choice (I
  like rosemary and thyme)
1 bay leaf
5 cloves garlic, slightly crushed with side
  of knife
Sea salt and pepper

Take the lamb out of the fridge, and allow it to come to room temperature (about 30 minutes). Preheat the oven to 350°F. Heat the fat of your choice in a Dutch oven, and sauté the vegetables for 5 minutes. Add the lamb, broth or stock, wine, herbs, bay leaf, and garlic, and cook, covered, in the oven for 3½ hours. (You can also transfer to a Crock-Pot and cook for 6 hours on low.) Season with sea salt and pepper. The lamb will be very tender and juicy. Remove the lamb and vegetables to a serving platter; conserve the drippings for the gravy.

GRAVY

2 cups lamb or beef stock
1 tablespoon gelatin
Sea salt and pepper

Follow the instructions for giblet gravy, page 76.

Note: *If you want something less involved, lamb chops are quick and easy. Just rub them with a little sea salt, pepper, garlic, ghee, and herbs of your choice. If you have time, let them sit and marinate for about 30 minutes; then throw them onto a hot grill or heavy-bottomed skillet for 3 to 4 minutes per side. Transfer to a 200°F oven for 10 to 15 minutes, depending on the thickness (for medium rare). Allow to rest for an additional 5 minutes. They are delicious and easy for kids to pick up and eat!*

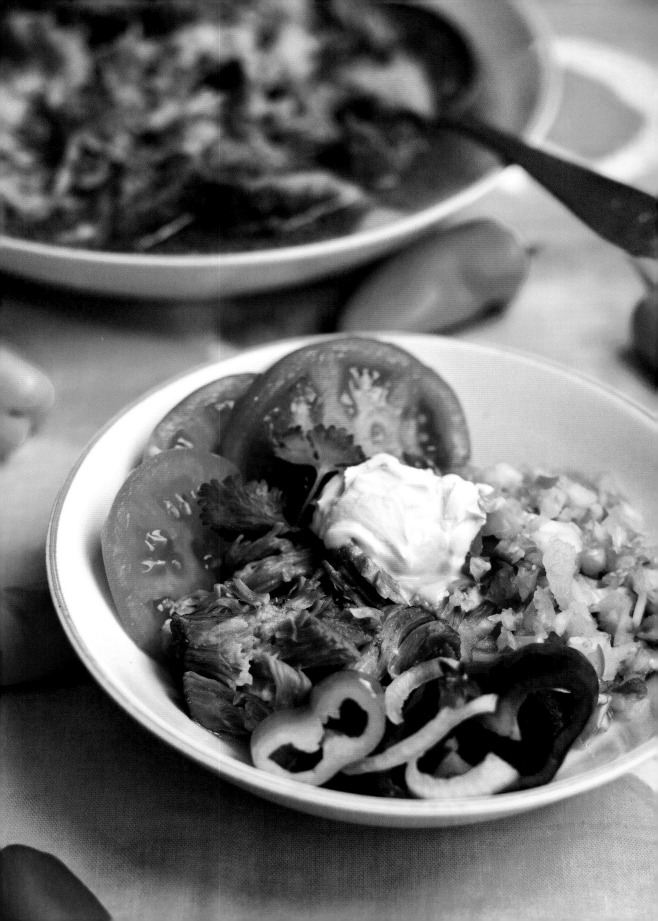

PORK CARNITAS
Serves 8 to 10

We often enjoy Pork Carnitas Mexican-style, with fermented hot sauce, salsa, cultured cream, cilantro . . . "The Works." But we also love this recipe with Mixed Roasted Peppers; Sweet, Spicy Caramelized Onions (recipes follow); and of course Lacto-Fermented BBQ Sauce (page 110)!

3 pounds boneless pork shoulder roast
1 teaspoon sea salt
1 teaspoon garlic powder
1 teaspoon ground cumin
½ teaspoon crumbled dried oregano
½ teaspoon ground coriander
¼ teaspoon cinnamon
2 cups chicken broth or stock
2 bay leaves

Cut the pork into five or six small pieces (your butcher will do this if you ask). Combine all of the spices in a bowl. Rub the spices all over the pork, and place the pieces in your slow cooker. Pour the broth on top, and drop in the bay leaves. A VitaClay will take 2 hours; a regular Crock-Pot will take 6 to 8 hours on low, or 5 to 6 hours on high.

Sweet, Spicy Caramelized Onions
Serves 4 to 6

3 tablespoons coconut oil, ghee,
   lard, or butter
3–4 white or red onions, sliced
1 tablespoon honey
Pinch of cayenne or dash or two of
   Hot Nicky (page 241)

In a frying pan, melt the fat of your choice and add the onion rings, separating the rings as you toss them in. Cook over medium-low heat, covered, for about 45 minutes, stirring occasionally to prevent sticking. When the onions are caramelized and golden, turn off the heat, add the honey and cayenne, and stir to incorporate.

Mixed Roasted Peppers
Serves 4 to 6

1 pound peppers: a mix of sweet and hot
   (bell, poblano, jalapeño)
Sea salt and pepper
2 tablespoons lard, ghee, coconut oil,
   or butter

Preheat the oven to 350 to 375°F. Place the peppers on a cookie sheet. Sprinkle with salt and pepper, and add dollops of fat. Place in the oven, let the fat melt for 2 or 3 minutes, and toss. This is a good way to avoid using a separate pan to melt the fat—in other words, a good way to cut back on dirty dishes. Roast for 1 hour, tossing a few times throughout.

RARE ROAST BEEF
Serves 8 to 10

Talk about a money saver. I went to Whole Foods the other day to buy cold cuts for my kids' lunches. I was bugged that the beef wasn't 100 percent grass-fed and that it was going to cost me $32 for 2 pounds of sliced roast beef! For pretty much the same price, I could buy a 4-pound, 100 percent grass-fed roast to cook myself. This was double the amount of meat, easy to make, and so tasty.

1 3- to 4-pound grass-fed roast beef
   (bottom or top round)
1 tablespoon garlic powder
1 teaspoon paprika
1 teaspoon black pepper
1 large onion, sliced into rings (optional)

Preheat the oven to 500°F. Cover the roast with the garlic powder, paprika, and pepper. Place half the onion rings in a roasting pan or a Dutch oven. Position the seasoned roast on top of them, then put the additional onions on top to lend flavor and keep the roast moist. Cook in the oven for 5 minutes per pound, then turn off the oven and leave the roast there (keeping the door shut) for an hour. Remove the roast, and tent with foil. Let it rest again for an additional 10 to 15 minutes to allow juices to distribute evenly. Slice thinly against the grain. Store in the fridge, and slice as needed throughout the week.

Note: *You can make a delicious gravy by adding beef broth to the pan drippings. Sprinkle in a little gelatin to thicken, then season with salt and pepper to taste. Scrape the drippings from the bottom of the pan with the back of a wooden spoon. Simmer for 4 to 5 minutes, adjust the seasoning, and pour over slices of roast beef. This makes an easy dinner, with enough leftovers for lunch!*

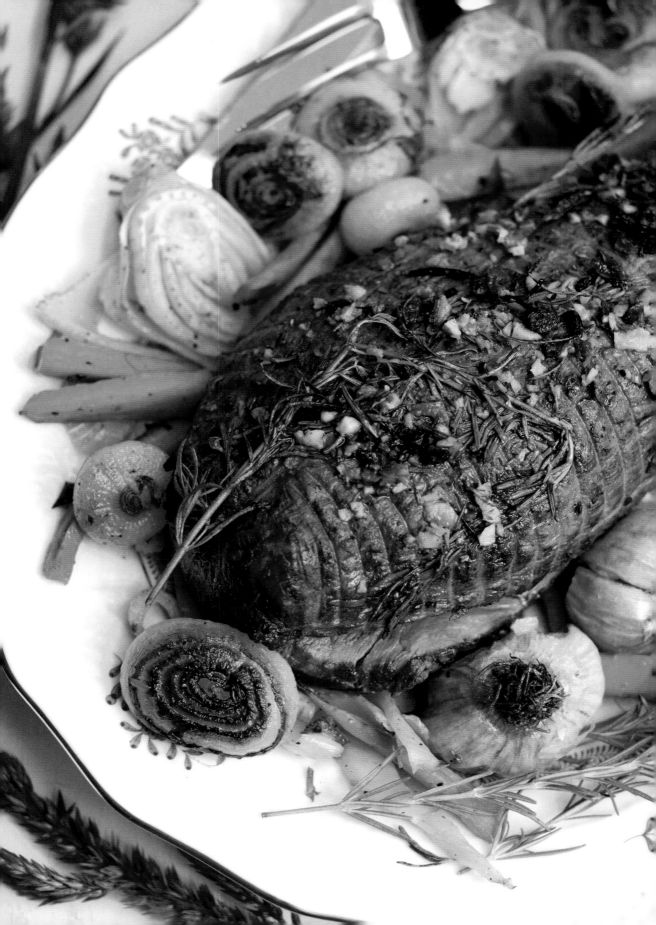

BEEF TENDERLOIN WITH PEARL ONIONS, HERBED BUTTER, AND ROASTED VEGETABLES
Serves 10 to 12

A few years ago, our neighbors served the most amazing beef tenderloin at their annual Christmas party. I emailed the host for his recipe, and he replied with the simplest instructions, as you will see. It calls for a more expensive cut of beef, but what a treat for a special occasion. A good meat thermometer makes things pretty foolproof! Thanks, Thayer!

If you have garlic lovers in the house, as I do, you can increase the number of garlic bulbs. Our kids love roasted garlic so much that no matter how much I cook, there is never enough.

5 pounds whole beef filet

4 bulbs garlic, for garnish

2–3 tablespoons beef tallow

3 cloves garlic, for rub

4–5 sprigs fresh rosemary (leave 2 or 3 whole sprigs to stuff under string)

2 pounds pearl onions (or sliced white onions)

Sea salt and pepper

Preheat the oven to 325°F. Take the beef out of the fridge, sprinkle it with salt and pepper, and allow it to come to room temperature, about 30 minutes.

Cut off the tops of the garlic bulbs (leaving the skins on and each bulb intact); place them on a piece of tinfoil (or in a garlic cooker). Pour a bit of melted fat over the top of each bulb and enclose in the tinfoil. Place in the oven for about 45 minutes to 1 hour, then set aside; maintain the oven temperature.

Place four or five pieces of string around the tenderloin to encourage it to cook uniformly (your butcher will do this for you if you ask). In an ovenproof pan over medium-high heat, brown the tenderloin in a bit of beef tallow, 2 to 3 minutes per side. Remove the meat to a plate. Warm more tallow in the pan. Finely chop the garlic cloves and two or three sprigs of the rosemary (leave the remainder whole); add to the warmed beef tallow, then spread the garlic, rosemary, and tallow mixture all over the tenderloin on the plate.

Place the tenderloin in a pan and scatter the onions around, sprinkling them with salt and pepper and a bit of fat. Cook in the hot oven for 30 minutes. (If you have a smaller cut, check for doneness earlier.) If you have a meat thermometer, cook until it reads 130 to 135°F (140°F is medium rare). Remove the tenderloin from the oven, and set it on a cutting board on the counter, uncovered, to rest and settle (about 20 minutes). It should be medium rare. Continue to cook the onions in the oven, if necessary, while the beef is resting. Slice the tenderloin and serve alongside the pearl onions with roasted vegetables of your choice (page 222), roasted garlic, and some nice herbed butter on top (page 123).

BURGERS THREE WAYS

We truly love burgers in our house . . . all different ways. The great thing about burgers is that you can customize your own toppings, and in our house we love our dips and sauces! My husband does not enjoy big chunks of anything in his burgers, but some of us love to mix it up here and there. If you can get your meat ground with the organs, even better! I often mix one pound with organs with one pound plain ground beef, and nobody knows the difference.

For the classic burger with any kind of meat, I just shape 1 pound of good room-temperature meat into six to eight patties and add salt and pepper before frying them in my cast-iron pan or throwing them on the grill. Cook for about 4 minutes per side for medium rare. Remove, and let rest for a few minutes. If you would like to add cheese, place under the broiler for an additional minute or throw a lid on the top of your cast-iron pan for a minute or two to gently melt the cheese.

To change things up a bit, try these different combinations, and remember that these all make good meatballs, too.

Beef Burgers
Serves 8

2 pounds grass-fed beef
Sea salt and pepper
1 red onion, chopped finely
4 teaspoons mustard
2 teaspoons coconut aminos (optional)
2 egg yolks

Delicious with fermented mayo, pickles, ketchup (page 110), and mustard (page 109). (See photo on page 177.)

Lamb Burgers
Serves 8

2 pounds ground lamb
1 teaspoon cinnamon
Pinch of paprika
1 red onion, minced
2 cloves garlic, minced

2 egg yolks
3 tablespoons chopped fresh mint or
   cilantro
Pinch of sea salt

Pork Burgers
Serves 8

2 pounds ground pork
1 red onion, minced
2 cloves garlic, minced
2 egg yolks
¼ cup chopped fresh sage, thyme,
   or parsley
2 tablespoons mustard
1 apple, shredded

These are delicious with Fermented Pear and Apple Chutney (page 90).

ROASTED PORK SAUSAGE WITH RED ONION AND BUTTERNUT SQUASH
Serves 4 to 6

I needed a quick dinner one night, and Debra, the owner of our neighborhood health food store, recommended a variation on this recipe. Serve it with a simple salad, and you are all set!

1 butternut squash, peeled, seeded, and cubed

2 red onions, cut into wedges

1 pound sausage, squeezed out of the casing and chopped into 1-inch pieces

Sea salt and pepper

2–3 tablespoons coconut oil, ghee, or animal fat

Preheat the oven to 350°F. On a cookie sheet, combine the squash, onions, and sausage. Season with salt and pepper, and add the fat. Place in the oven for 5 minutes to melt the fat, then toss to coat everything. Roast for 45 to 50 minutes, or until the squash is soft. Easy!

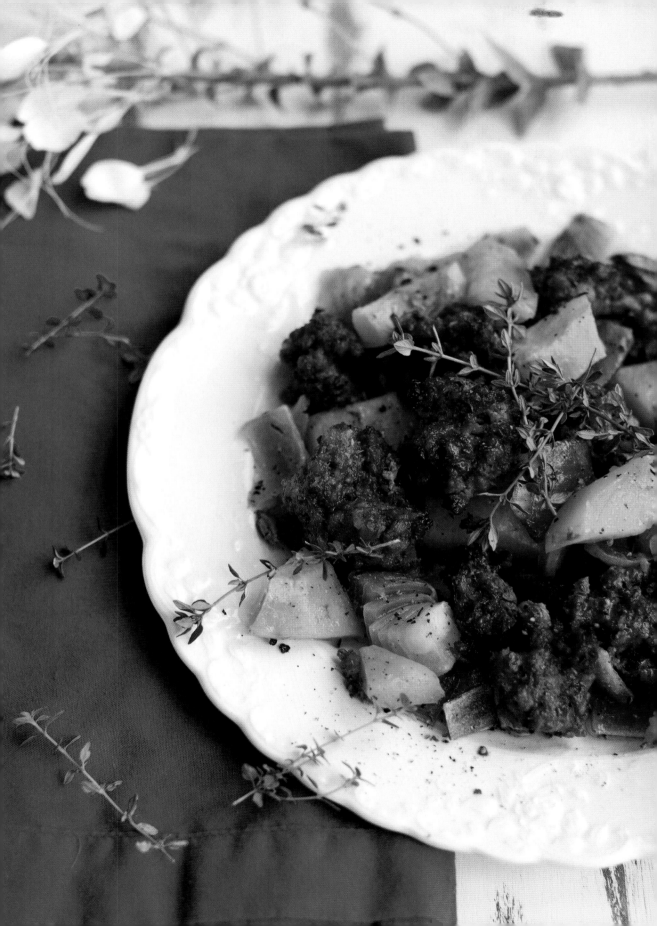

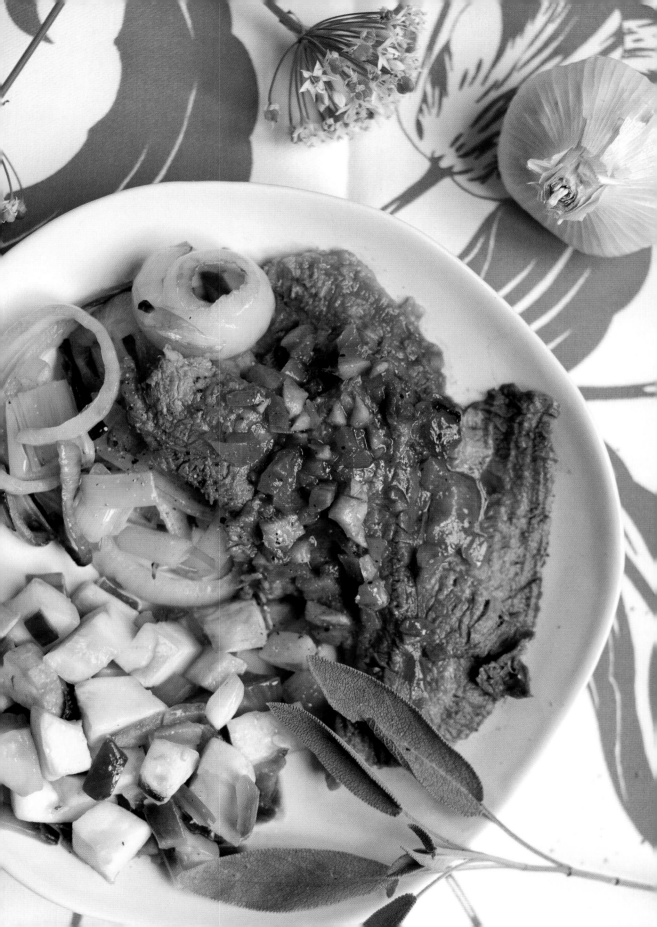

MOM'S MARINATED FLANK STEAK
Serves 4 to 6

Growing up, one of my favorite dinners was my mom's flank steak. Now my own kids love it, and I double the recipe so we can enjoy leftovers for lunch. Flank steak, hanger steak, and skirt steak are all reasonably priced options. This marinade also works well for pork tenderloin with red onions and sliced tart apples.

¼ cup ghee, tallow, or palm oil (you can use olive oil, too, but wipe it off before cooking as its smoke point is not very high)

¼ cup honey (optional)

2½ teaspoons ground ginger or 2–3 inches freshly grated gingerroot

Juice of 1 lime

¼ cup coconut aminos

1 tablespoon apple cider vinegar

½ onion, finely diced

2 cloves garlic, pressed or finely chopped

2 pounds steak

Sea salt and pepper

Mix all of the ingredients (except the steak, salt, and pepper) in a bowl. Place the meat in a glass dish. Pour the marinade over, and swish around to make sure all parts of the steak are coated. Cover, and place in the fridge for at least 3 hours and up to 2 days, turning every so often. The oils will get hard in the fridge, so be sure to bring the meat to room temperature before cooking.

Season your grill! Before firing it up, soak a paper towel with coconut oil or lard, and rub it along the clean grates. This will ensure that the steak doesn't stick. Preheat the grill to high heat.

Generously salt and pepper both sides of your steak. Place on the grill for 4 to 6 minutes per side (you can also cook it under the broiler for 4 to 5 minutes per side if you don't have a grill handy). Remove, place on your cutting board, tent with tinfoil to keep the heat in, and let it rest for 10 minutes. Flank steak is best cooked medium rare—pink in the middle. Open your hand, palm facing down, and feel the fleshy skin between your thumb and index finger; that is what a medium rare steak will feel like. The tip of your nose is well done, and that will make for a very tough steak. Slice thinly against the grain on a diagonal, and serve. You can gently boil the remaining marinade for 7 to 10 minutes and use as a sauce to pour over steak.

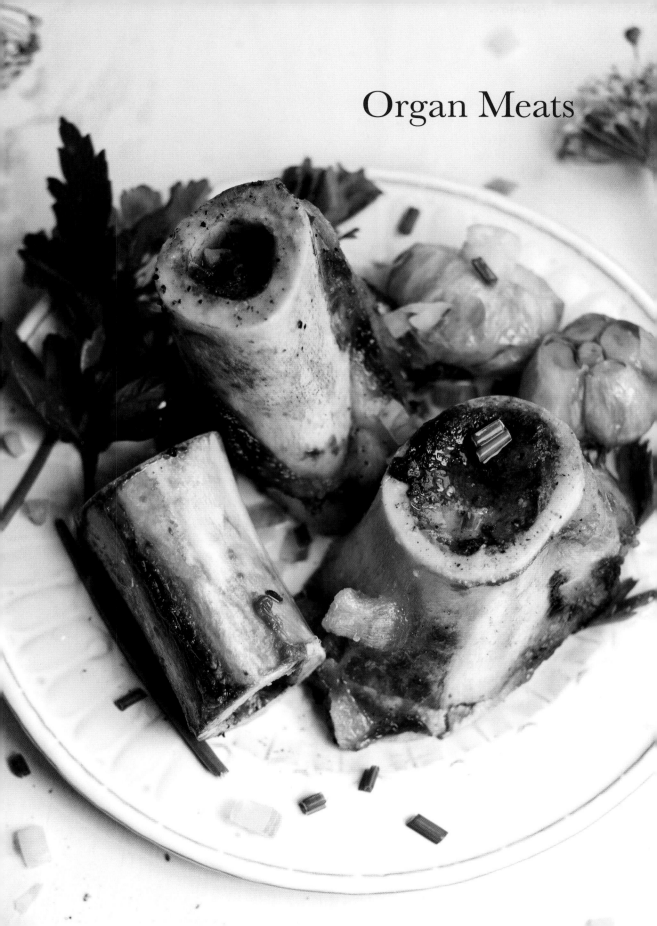

Organ Meats

Why eat organ meats? Sally Fallon Morell explains in *Nourishing Traditions*:

> Compared with muscle meats, organ meats are richer in just about every nutrient, including minerals like phosphorus, iron, copper, magnesium and iodine, and in B vitamins including B_1, B_2, B_6, folic acid and especially vitamin B_{12}. Organ meats provide high levels of the all-important fat-soluble vitamins A, D, E, and K, especially if the animals live outside in the sunlight and eat green grass. Organ meats are also rich in beneficial fatty acids such as arachidonic acid, EPA and DHA. Organ meats even contain vitamin C—liver is richer in vitamin C than apples or carrots! Even if you add only small amounts of organ meats to your ground meat dishes, you are providing your family with super nutrition . . . in ways that everyone likes and are easy to consume.

MEAT LOAF WITH ORGANS
Serves 6 to 8

I am fortunate to have a farmer (Miller's Organic Farm; see resources) who will grind the organs right into the meat for me, which makes life easier. If you don't have that option, place ½ of organ meat in your food processor, pulse ten times to break up, then mix by hand into your ground meat.

1½ pounds ground meat (beef, pastured lamb, pork, or a combination)
½ pound ground organs (chicken or beef liver and/or heart)
3 pastured eggs
1 small red onion, finely diced
3 cloves garlic, minced
1 teaspoon sea salt
1 teaspoon dried oregano
1 teaspoon dried thyme
1 cup button mushrooms or baby portobellos, chopped fine (optional)
1 cup finely grated carrot (optional)
1 teaspoon fresh cracked pepper
1 tablespoon kelp seasoning (optional, but great for trace minerals)
8–10 slices bacon (optional)

Preheat the oven to 350°F. Place all of the ingredients (except the bacon) in a bowl, and mix together with your hands. Place the mixture into a glass loaf pan and lay strips of bacon across the top. Bake for 1 hour, or until the center reaches 160°F. You can enjoy the meat loaf right away, or freeze it in thick slices for quick school lunches. I often double the recipe and stick a whole uncooked loaf in the freezer for a fast future dinner. Just wrap in parchment paper, then tinfoil, and pop into the freezer.

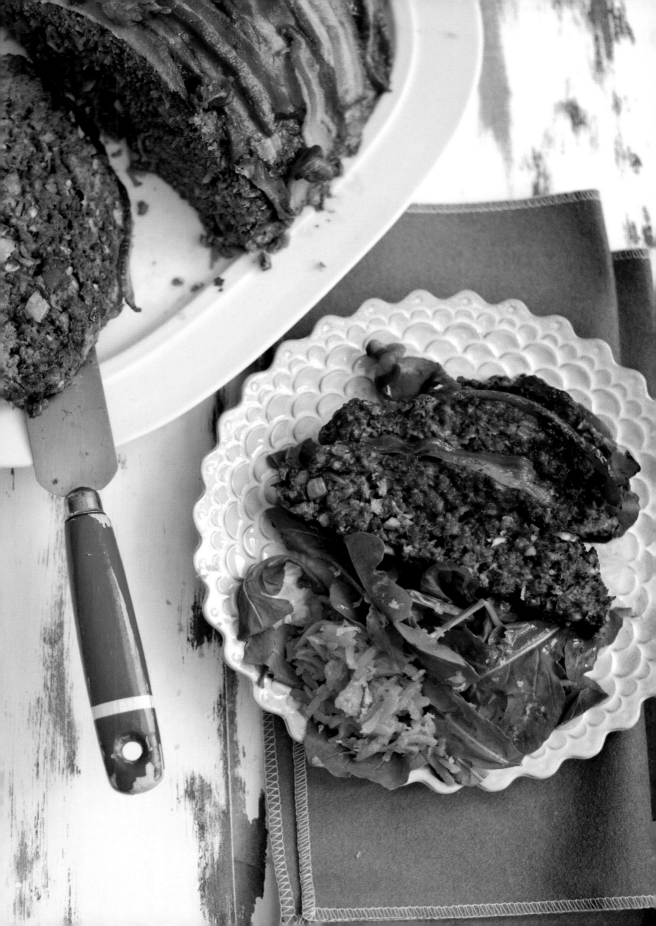

CHICKEN AND LIVER "ENCHILADAS"
Serves 6 to 8

I have adapted this from a friend's delicious recipe for enchiladas. My kids all love it, so it's an easy way to get liver into them. And nobody ever complains about the mysteriously absent tortillas . . .

Sauce

25 tomatillos
1 poblano pepper
1 cup chicken broth or stock
2–3 cloves garlic
1½ bunches cilantro

2 handfuls baby spinach
Juice of ½ lime
2 whole scallions
Sea salt and pepper

Meat "Filling"

2 whole chicken breasts or 12–16 bone-
    less chicken thighs
½–1 pound chicken livers
3 cups chicken broth or stock
1 cup dry white wine
1 scallion
Sea salt and pepper
1–2 cups grated raw cheddar cheese
    (optional)

To make the sauce, preheat the oven to 400°F. Remove the husks from the tomatillos and wash (these are a little sticky, but don't worry). Roast them on a cookie sheet until brown, about 30 to 45 minutes. Let cool, and place in a blender. Add the remaining sauce ingredients, and blend until smooth. Pour into a saucepan over medium-low heat, and simmer until the sauce starts to deepen in color, about 15 minutes (this is easy to make and freeze, so in the summer months gather what you can and enjoy all winter). Reduce the oven temperature to 350°F.

To make the "filling," place the chicken and livers in a pot with the broth or stock, wine, scallion, salt, and pepper. Poach for about 15 minutes; shred the chicken, then mash the livers. Add the chicken and livers to a casserole dish, and pour the sauce over the top. Place in the now 350°F oven for 30 minutes. Toward the end of baking time, sprinkle shredded raw cheese on top, and gently melt.

Serve with cultured cream (page 30), chopped tomatoes, cilantro, and guacamole (page 116).

CHICKEN LIVERS WRAPPED IN BACON
Serves 4 to 6

I don't remember having many organ meats other than these chicken livers as a small child. They must have made a quick meal for my mother to prepare. But when convenience foods came in, organs apparently went out. Still, Mom fondly reminisces about the "liver parties" of her summers in Maine as a young adult . . . can you imagine? I think we should bring them back into style!

1 pound chicken livers, cleaned and cut into 2-inch pieces
1 pound nitrite/nitrate- and sugar-free bacon (see resources)

Preheat the oven to 350°F. Wrap each chicken liver with ½ piece of bacon, and hold together with a toothpick. Place on a parchment-lined cookie sheet, and bake for 15 minutes or until the bacon is crisp. Place on a platter and serve.

SWEET LIVER AND ONIONS
Serves 4 to 6

Our German babysitter suggested this recipe for liver and onions. It is delicious and definitely makes liver easier to swallow for those who are not fans.

8 slices nitrite/nitrate- and sugar-free bacon (see resources)
¼ cup unsalted butter or fat of choice, divided
2 large onions, sliced
3 apples, cored and cut into eighths
2 tablespoons coconut vinegar
¼ cup dry white wine
1 teaspoon honey
1 calf's liver, washed, dried, and cut into bite-sized pieces
Juice of 1 lemon
½ bunch fresh parsley, chopped, for garnish
Sea salt and pepper

Preheat the oven to 350°F. Place the bacon on a cookie sheet, and set in the oven until crisp, 10 to 15 minutes. Reserve the bacon for garnish.

Pour a few tablespoons of the bacon grease into a skillet over medium heat, and add a tablespoon of the butter. Sauté the onions in the fat, stirring occasionally, until they are soft. Add the apples, and cook for another 5 minutes. Add the vinegar and the wine, and bring the mixture to a boil. Boil for a few minutes, allowing the mixture to thicken a bit. Turn off the heat and stir in the honey. Set aside.

In a clean skillet, heat the remaining 3 tablespoons butter and add the liver. Sauté the liver for 3 to 4 minutes, turning occasionally, until it's browned and slightly pink in the middle. Add the liver to the apple mixture, and squeeze fresh lemon juice on top. Remove to a serving bowl or platter, and garnish by crumbling the reserved bacon and sprinkling it on top, along with the chopped parsley. Season with salt and pepper to taste. Crumbled raw blue cheese or Gorgonzola makes a wonderful addition if desired.

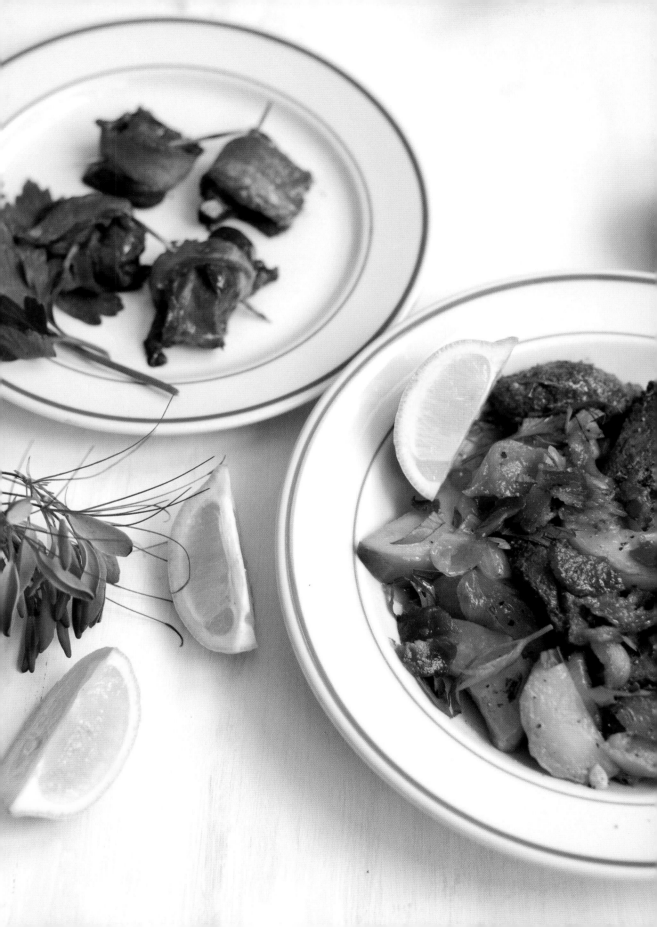

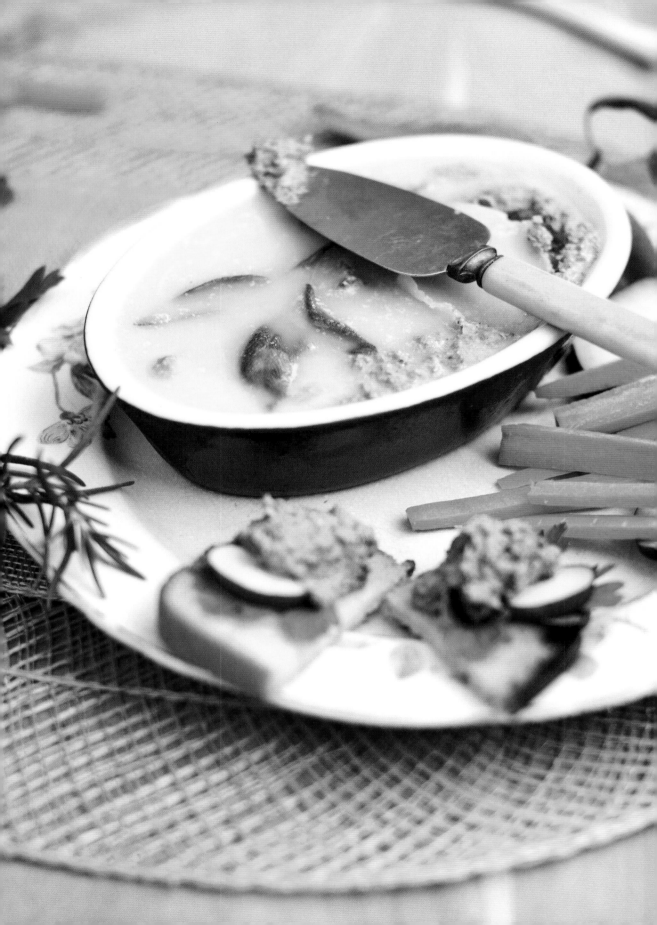

CHICKEN LIVER PÂTÉ
Serves 8 to 10

The first pâté recipe I ever made was from Sally Fallon Morell's book *Nourishing Traditions*. I have pretty much stuck with it, as it's delicious and easy to make.

3 tablespoons butter

1 pound chicken or duck livers, or a combination

1 bunch green onions, chopped

½ pound mushrooms, washed, dried, and coarsely chopped

1 clove garlic, chopped

⅔ cup dry white wine

½ teaspoon dry mustard

1 tablespoon lemon juice

¼ teaspoon dried dill

¼ teaspoon dried rosemary

¼ cup butter, softened (plus a little additional for melting on top)

Sea salt

Melt 3 tablespoons of butter in a heavy skillet. Add the livers, onions, and mushrooms and cook, stirring occasionally, for about 10 minutes, until the livers are browned. Add the garlic, wine, mustard, lemon juice, and herbs. Bring to a boil and cook, uncovered, until the liquid is gone. Allow to cool. Process in a food processor with ¼ cup of softened butter. Season to taste. Place in a crock or mold, pour a little extra melted butter on top to preserve, cover with plastic wrap, and chill well. I often divide this into four ramekins and freeze individually.

MEXICAN CHICKEN HEARTS
Serves 6 to 8

Okay, I have to admit, this was the *very* last recipe I made and tested for this book. I was, well, not so keen on hearts, I guess. But I knew I wanted to provide more organ meat options, so as Kelly the Kitchen Kop once said, "It was time to put my big girl panties on, and just try it." When I did, once again I was pleasantly surprised: My whole family actually tucked into a meal of . . . chicken hearts! Who knew? The lesson learned here is to not make the same mistake our parents made. Give your kids organ meat from the beginning, and it will become their "norm." This is another recipe inspired by Deborah Krasner.

1 pound chicken hearts

2 chile peppers, with seeds (remove the seeds if you want less spice)

4 cloves garlic

1 teaspoon cumin

1 teaspoon coriander

½ teaspoon sea salt

½ teaspoon pepper

¼ cup filtered water

½ cup coconut aminos

2 tablespoons animal fat or ghee

2 onions, sliced

2 bell peppers (any color), finely diced

1 pound fresh tomatoes, chopped, or
   1 jar or can (28 ounces) diced tomatoes

Slice the hearts in half, and in half again, rinse them in a colander, drain, and remove the aortas (I forgot to do this the first time, and they were still delicious; it's just more appetizing to look at when valves are removed). Place the chile peppers and three of the garlic cloves in a food processor. Process to a very fine dice, and set the mixture aside. Put the hearts in a medium-sized bowl, and add the cumin, coriander, salt, pepper, and remaining garlic clove, chopped. Stir around, cover, and place in the fridge to marinate for 30 minutes or longer. In another bowl, add the water, coconut aminos, and some fresh cracked pepper. Meanwhile, melt the fat in a large frying pan over medium-high heat, and add the chile-garlic paste. Sauté for about 30 seconds, then add the onions. Cook for an additional 2 to 3 minutes, and add hearts. Stir to cover the hearts with the marinade until they become colored and almost cooked through, 1 to 2 minutes. Add the coconut amino mixture, the

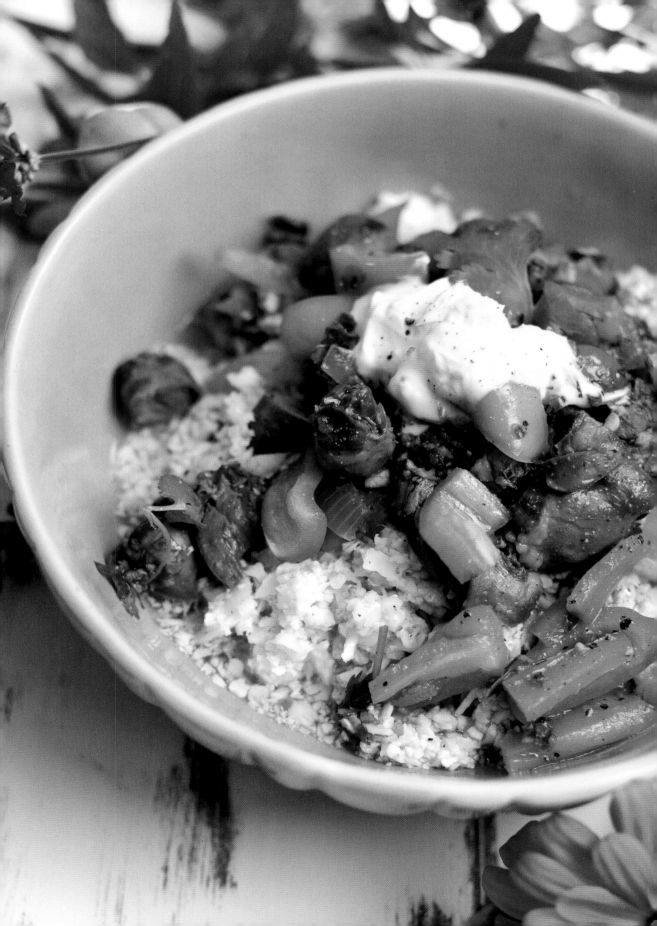

diced bell peppers, and the chopped tomatoes. Season with more salt and pepper, then cover and cook for an additional 5 minutes. Serve in a bowl as is or—even better—over cauliflower rice (page 87).

ROASTED BONE MARROW
Serves 4 to 6

I never thought I'd be roasting bone marrow, but I'm glad I finally did. Bone marrow is a great source of minerals and calcium. It's particularly wonderful for pregnant or nursing moms, or women who are trying to get pregnant. It is very, very nutrient-dense. I remember trying bone marrow at a restaurant several years back—I must admit, I was squeamish about it. What a pleasant surprise! It was lovely, rich, and satisfying. Now my kids enjoy it, too. In particular, my kids devour the roasted garlic, so I always make extra.

3 bulbs garlic

2 tablespoons ghee or animal fat (for garlic bulbs)

6–10 marrow bones (3–4 inches apiece; your butcher will slice a longer piece lengthwise upon request)

Pinch of sea salt and fresh cracked pepper

Juice of 1 lemon

Fresh parsley, chopped, for garnish

Toast or crackers, for serving (I usually crisp up some Coconut Butter Bread, page 118, in the toaster oven and cut it into squares)

Preheat the oven to 400°F. Cut off the tops of the garlic bulbs and pour some melted animal fat or ghee on top. Wrap the bulbs in foil or put them in a garlic roaster, and place in the oven for 1 hour. Remove and set aside.

Place the marrow bones, standing upward (or lying flat if cut lengthwise), in a heavy pan or rimmed cookie sheet, and sprinkle with salt and pepper. Roast for about 30 minutes, being careful not to overcook and have all the fat run out of the bone. You can tell when it's finished if there's a crust and the marrow separates from the bone a bit. Remove from the oven, and squeeze fresh lemon juice over the top; be sure to drizzle any fat that has melted out over the top as well. Sprinkle with parsley. Serve on toast with the roasted garlic (feel free to squeeze out the garlic beforehand or allow your guests to pick them out individually). Fermented Fig Jam (page 237) is a nice addition, if you want to be a little fancier or entice your kiddos to try it! (See photo on page 195.)

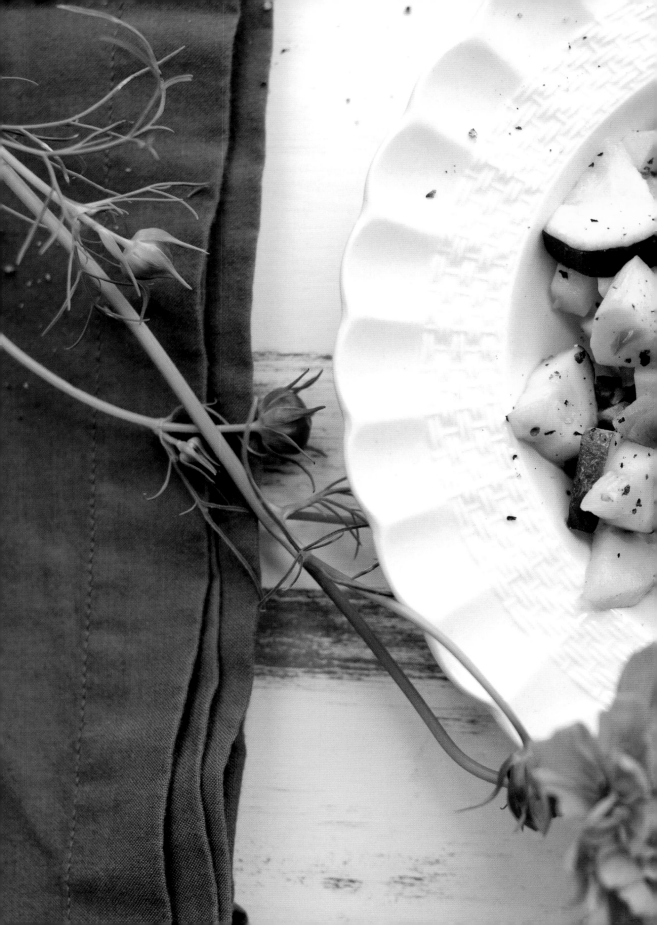

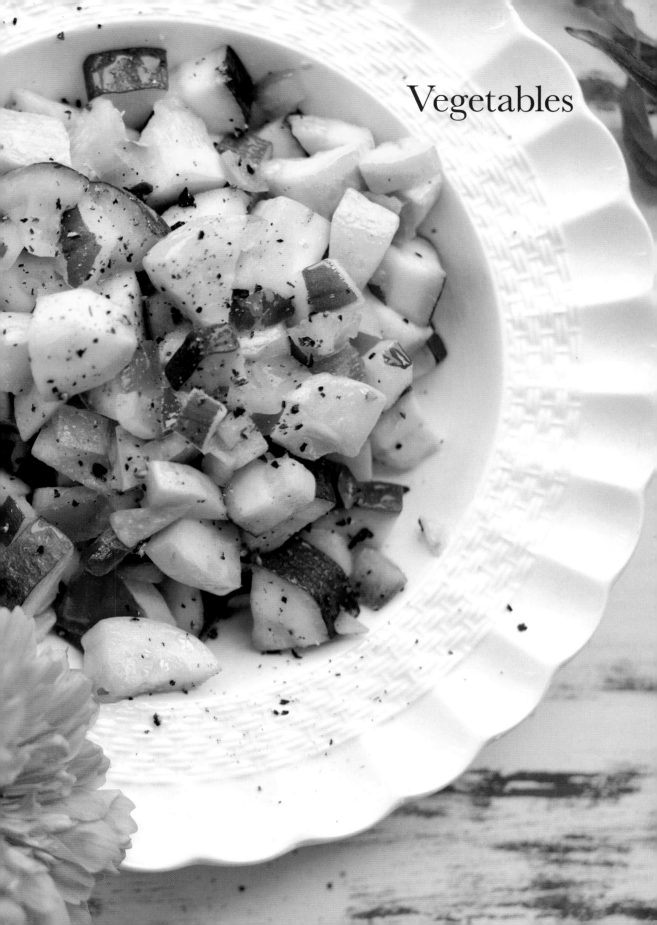

Vegetables

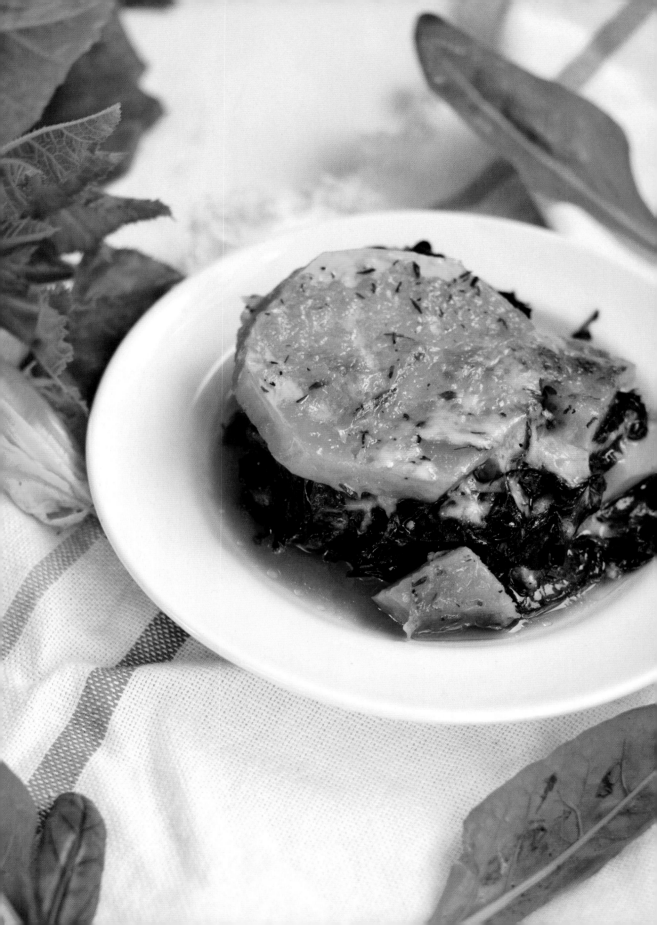

BUTTERNUT SQUASH AND SWISS CHARD LASAGNA

Serves 6 to 8 as a main course, or 10 to 12 as a side

You can also scale this recipe up by 50 percent if you're serving a crowd. Feel free to substitute kale for the chard or use a mixture of both.

I always make this in two versions: one with cheese and butter, and one without for our daughter. It is equally good without the cheese. For her I use pastured lard or bacon grease, as she can't eat dairy. You can also make it without the sausage if you would prefer it as a side to a meat or fish dish. It takes a little bit of assembly time, but it is well worth it!

1 large or 2 small butternut squash, peeled, seeded, and sliced ⅛ inch thick
Sea salt and pepper
3 tablespoons butter, cut into pieces or fat of choice
1–2 large bunches Swiss chard, chopped (leave out stems, if you wish)
1–2 cups cooked ground sausage
2–3 tablespoons dried thyme
1½–2 cups grated cheddar (optional), divided
1–2 cups chicken broth
½ cup grated Parmesan (optional)

Preheat the oven to 350°F. Grease a 9 by 13-inch baking dish. Layer a third of the squash slices on the bottom of the pan; season with salt, pepper, and a little chopped butter. Top with half the chard; add a layer of sausage, a big pinch of thyme, and more salt, pepper, and butter. Add a third of the cheese. Top with half of the remaining squash, then all the remaining chard, salt, pepper, butter, and thyme, and another layer of sausage. Add half the cheddar, then finish with the last of the squash.

Carefully pour the broth over the dish. It'll seem very full, but don't worry: It cooks down. Cover tightly with foil, and bake for an hour. Carefully remove from oven, and take off the foil. Top the lasagna with the remaining cheddar and the Parmesan. Broil until the cheese is melted and golden.

BRUSSELS SPROUTS WITH BACON
Serves 4 to 6

My good friend Suzy shared this recipe with me, and it is, hands down, our family's favorite way to have brussels sprouts!

1 pound brussels sprouts
½ pound nitrite/nitrate- and sugar-free bacon; or more if your kids are like mine (see resources)
1 tablespoon stone-ground mustard
1 tablespoon honey
Sea salt and pepper

Rinse and trim the brussels sprouts and cut them in half. Cook the bacon in a large skillet on the stovetop or bake on a cookie sheet in a 350°F oven for 15 minutes.

While the bacon is cooking, blanch the brussels sprouts: Plunge them into boiling water for about 2 minutes until they turn bright green, then transfer to an ice-cold water bath.

When the bacon is finished, transfer it to cutting board, reserving the grease as well. In a skillet, add the brussels sprouts to the bacon grease. Add the mustard, and cook on medium for about another 5 minutes until soft enough to eat. Turn off the heat and gently stir in honey. Coarsely chop the bacon, scatter it on top of the sprouts, season with salt and pepper, and serve.

This recipe can easily be doubled!

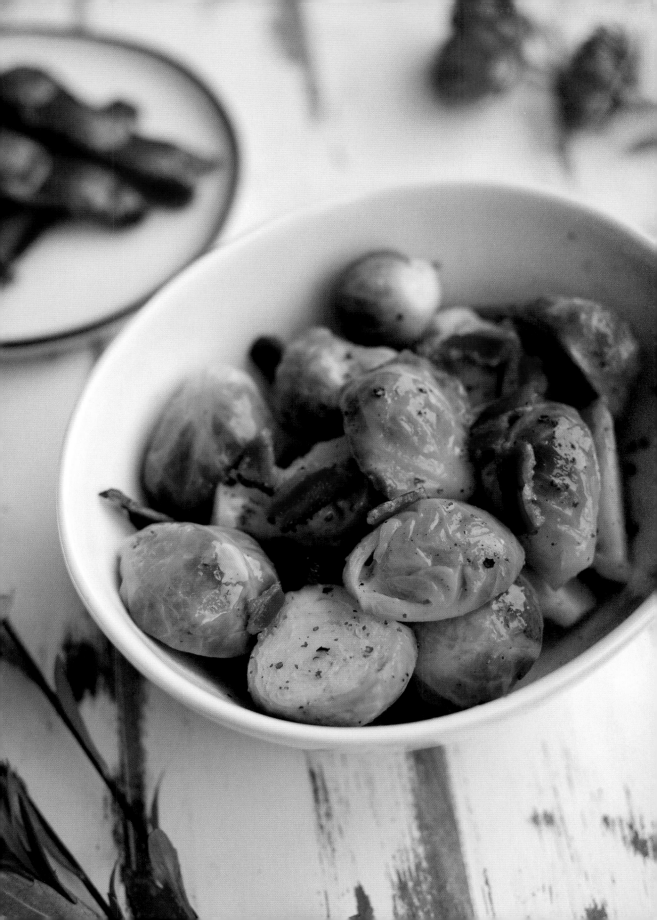

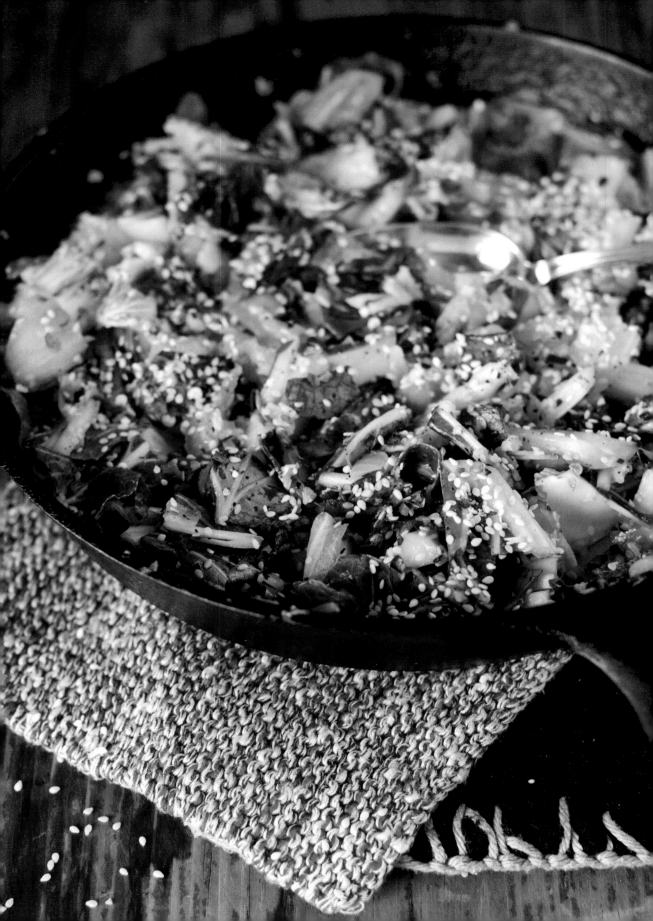

GINGER BOK CHOY
Serves 6 to 8

This is another great recipe inspired by my CSA farmers. Bok choy is especially tender and tasty when harvested fresh. Look for it at your local farmers' market.

1 head bok choy
1 small yellow onion, chopped
2 tablespoons sesame oil
5 cloves garlic, minced
1 small piece of gingerroot, chopped fine
1 tablespoon coconut aminos
1 teaspoon hot pepper flakes (optional)
Sea salt and pepper
2 tablespoons sesame seeds, for garnish

Chop the bok choy into 1-inch pieces, separating the green tops from the white bottoms. Sauté the onion in the sesame oil for about 5 minutes until tender. Add the white bottoms of the bok choy, and sauté for an additional 5 minutes. Add the green tops, garlic, ginger, coconut aminos, and hot pepper flakes. Stir to incorporate, then cook for another few minutes. Add salt and pepper to taste and garnish with sesame seeds.

GREEN PEAS WITH SHALLOTS AND BACON
Serves 4 to 6

¼ pound nitrite/nitrate- and sugar-free
   bacon (see resources)
1 shallot, diced
1 pound fresh shelled peas, or
   1 bag frozen organic peas
Sea salt and pepper

Preheat the oven to 350°F. Place the bacon on a cookie sheet, and bake for 15 minutes or until crisp. Set aside. Pour 1 tablespoon of the bacon grease into a skillet over medium heat (the remaining grease can be discarded), and add the shallot. Sauté until translucent, then add the peas. Stir gently for 3 to 6 minutes, or until heated through. Season with salt and pepper. Transfer to a bowl, and crumble the bacon on top.

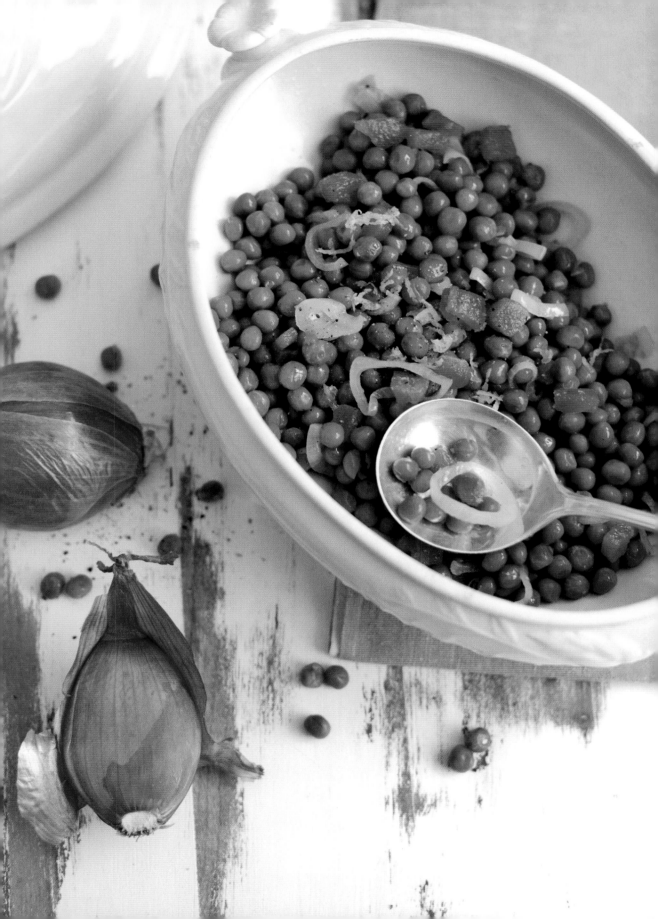

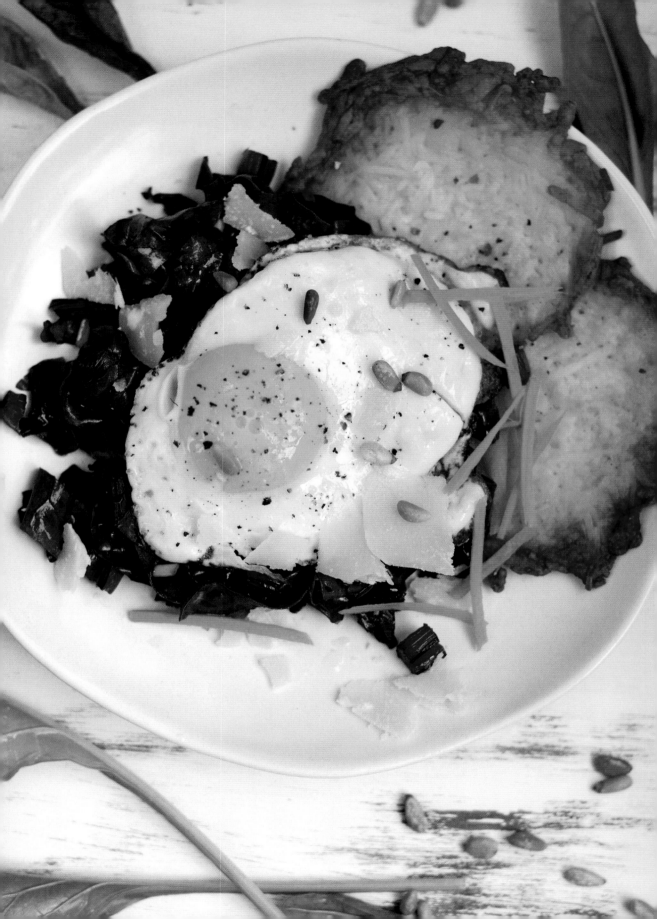

BEAUTIFUL CHARD
Serves 2 to 4

This makes a delicious and quick breakfast, lunch, or dinner!

2 tablespoons coconut oil or lard, divided
1 bunch chard, chopped (stems, too, if
   you wish)
3 cloves garlic, minced
1 teaspoon coconut vinegar
Handful of pine nuts, gently toasted
Sea salt and pepper
4 eggs
½ cup grated hard Italian cheese (such
   as raw Parmesan)
Olive oil, for serving

Heat 1 tablespoon of the fat in a large frying pan, add the chopped chard stems (if using), and sauté for 5 minutes. Add the garlic, and sauté for 2 minutes. Add the chard leaves, and cook until tender, about 5 more minutes. Add the vinegar and pine nuts, and cook for 1 minute more. Season with salt and pepper, and transfer to a serving dish.

Fry the eggs in the remaining tablespoon of fat. To serve, pile the chard on a plate, place an egg on top, and sprinkle with some shredded raw cheese. Give it a drizzle of olive oil, and season with salt and pepper to taste. Serve with Parmesan Crisps (page 247) and Ginger Carrots (page 235) or your ferment of choice.

PORTOBELLO PARMESAN
Serves 4 to 6

This is one dish I never expected my kids to eat, especially the non-mushroom-lovers. But somehow, this recipe makes mushroom lovers out of all of them! Inspired by Giada De Laurentiis.

3 tablespoons pastured lard or
   coconut oil
4–6 portobello mushrooms
½ teaspoon sea salt
¼ teaspoon freshly ground black pepper
2 cups Ed Giobbi's Sweet Marinara Sauce
   (page 116), or other tomato sauce
   of choice
½ cup shredded cheddar or Monterey
   Jack cheese
¼ cup grated Parmesan
2 tablespoons butter, cut into
   small pieces

Preheat the oven to 350°F. Drizzle fat over both sides of the mushrooms and onto the grill pan to prevent sticking. Season the mushrooms with salt and pepper, and grill them over medium-high heat until they are heated through and tender (about 5 minutes per side). Spread half the marinara sauce on the bottom of a 9 by 13-inch baking dish. Place the mushrooms in the pan (gills facing up), and top with the remaining marinara sauce. Sprinkle with a mix of the two cheeses, and top with butter pieces. Bake until the cheese melts and the top is golden brown, about 15 minutes. Serve with a nice salad.

SPAGHETTI SQUASH WITH OLIVE OIL AND BASIL
Serves 6 to 8

1 spaghetti squash
2–3 tablespoons butter, or ghee
1 clove garlic, pressed
Sea salt and pepper
Handful of fresh basil, chopped (add
   additional fresh herbs if you desire)
2 tablespoons olive oil
Handful of pine nuts
Raw Parmesan, shredded (optional)

Preheat the oven to 375°F. Cut the spaghetti squash in half lengthwise, and scoop out any seeds. Place the squash facedown on a cookie sheet with enough water to cover the bottom. Cover with aluminum foil, and cook for 45 minutes, or until a fork pierces right through the squash. Remove it from the oven and let it cool a bit. Scoop out the squash meat, using a fork to shred it into spaghetti-like strands.

Melt the fat in a pan on the stove, and add the spaghetti squash, garlic, salt, pepper, and fresh herbs. Gently stir to combine and heat through. Serve with a drizzle of fresh olive oil and pine nuts, or try a pesto (page 114) or Ed Giobbi's Marinara Sauce (page 116) for a more traditional spaghetti-like experience. Sprinkle Parmesan on top to garnish.

ROASTED ANYTHING
Serves 6 to 8

I used to roast vegetables in olive oil at 400 to 425°F for years . . . Yikes! Now I know better and keep delicate olive oil for salads or maybe a little light sautéing. Use the more heat-stable oils for roasting. Here is a list of the smoke points, also known as the burn points, for the various healthy fats I cook with. Remember, when you burn fat by heating it above its smoke point you are creating free radicals, which are best avoided.

Smoke Point for Fats

Unrefined coconut oil	350°F / 177°C	Duck fat	375°F / 191°C
Butter	350°F / 177°C	Tallow	400–420°F / 204–216°C
Lard	370°F / 188°C	Palm oil	450°F / 232°C
Schmaltz	375°F / 191°C	Ghee	485°F / 252°C

I do like to roast vegetables for my kids, and I use a basic formula for pretty much everything: 2 to 3 pounds vegetables, 2 to 4 tablespoons fat (duck fat is my favorite), and a few pinches of sea salt and fresh cracked pepper. I then add the extra spices I desire and throw it all into a 375°F oven for 30 to 45 minutes, tossing a few times throughout. Here are some of the combos I love . . . think of the frittatas you can make with the leftovers!

- Roasted cauliflower with herbes de Provence, sea salt, and pepper
- Roasted beets with rosemary, sea salt, and pepper
- Roasted zucchini and summer squash with Parmesan, sea salt, and pepper
- Roasted carrots with cumin, sea salt, and pepper
- Roasted butternut squash with red onion, sausage, rosemary, sea salt, and pepper (makes a great meal with a side salad)
- Roasted asparagus with lemon zest and a little Parmesan cheese on top, plus sea salt and pepper
- Roasted summer tomatoes, quartered, with red onion, garlic, and loads of fresh herbs: Puree into a sauce and freeze, adding sea salt and pepper upon reheating
- Roasted cherry tomatoes with garlic, basil, sea salt, and pepper
- Roasted eggplant with any color peppers, red onions, and garlic—eat as is or add a little tomato paste, olive oil, sea salt, and pepper, then puree into a dip
- Roasted broccoli with garlic, lemon zest, sea salt, and pepper
- Roasted brussels sprouts with bacon, sea salt, and pepper

- Roasted spaghetti squash with sea salt, butter, and fresh cracked pepper
- Roasted delicata squash with duck fat, sea salt, and pepper
- Roasted rutabaga or squash fries in duck fat with a little rosemary, sea salt, and pepper . . . yum!

SUMMER SQUASH SUCCOTASH
Serves 4 to 6

This recipe is especially handy for the summer months, when you have summer squash and zucchini coming out of your ears! It couldn't be easier, and the leftovers are delicious in a Frittata (page 77).

1–2 tablespoons coconut oil, ghee, or animal fat

2–4 summer squash and/or zucchini

1 red or white onion, chopped (red is prettier)

1 clove garlic, chopped

Sea salt and pepper

Handful of chopped parsley (optional)

Warm the fat in a skillet, and add the chopped zucchini and summer squash, along with the onion. Sauté for about 15 minutes, until soft. Add the garlic, salt, and pepper, and cook for an additional 5 minutes. Toss with the parsley and serve. (See photo on page 208.)

GRILLED EGGPLANT WITH BASIL AND PINE NUTS
Serves 4 to 6

Thanks to the countless hours I spent watching the Food Network while feeding babies nearly ten years ago, this dish was inspired by Giada De Laurentiis. It looks beautiful, tastes delicious, and is a total crowd pleaser!

3 tablespoons ghee or coconut oil
1–2 large eggplants or 5–6 small Japanese eggplants, sliced into ½-inch-wide slices (you can also substitute zucchini and/or summer squash)
Sea salt
½ cup lightly toasted pine nuts
⅓ cup herbed yogurt or kefir cheese (optional) (page 32)
¼ cup thinly sliced or torn fresh basil
3 tablespoons extra-virgin olive oil
Pepper

Place a grill pan over medium-high heat, or preheat a gas or charcoal grill.

Melt the ghee or coconut oil, and drizzle it over the slices of eggplant. Lightly salt the eggplant, and grill until tender and grill marks appear, 3 to 4 minutes per side.

Place the eggplant on a serving platter, and sprinkle with the pine nuts, yogurt cheese, and basil. Drizzle with extra-virgin olive oil and a pinch of sea salt and fresh cracked pepper.

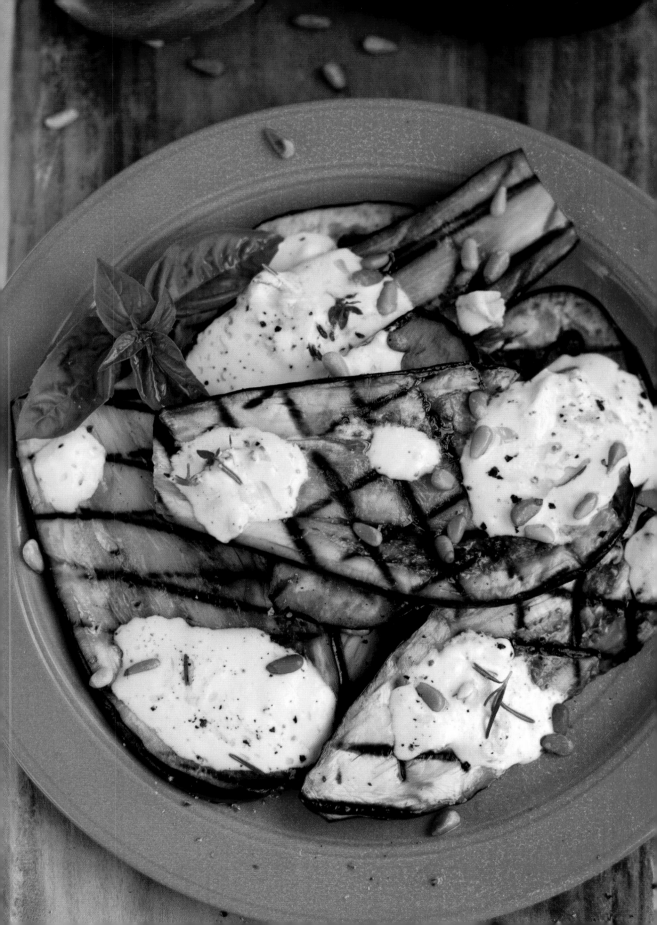

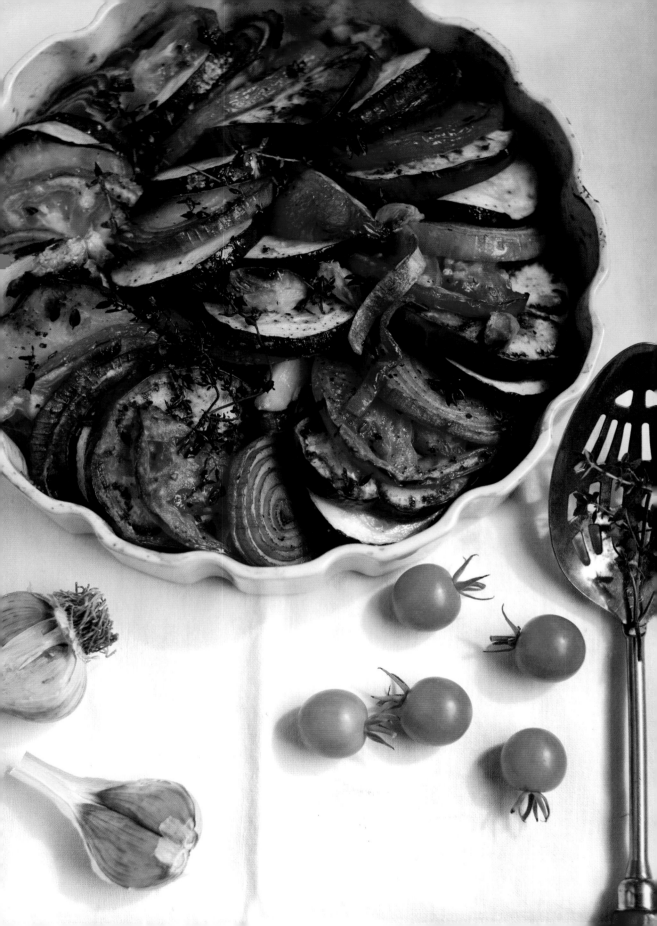

VEGETABLE TIAN
Serves 6 to 8

This simple but elegant dish is perfect for serving when company comes over and makes an especially nice side for fish. It's always beautiful, and the vegetables are completely interchangeable, so use what you have.

1 eggplant, sliced
1 red onion, sliced
1 zucchini, sliced
2 tomatoes, sliced
3 tablespoons ghee or fat of choice
1 teaspoon sea salt
½ teaspoon fresh cracked pepper
Handful of fresh thyme,
    stripped off stems
3 cloves garlic, smashed or chopped

Preheat the oven to 425°F. Place the vegetables in a big bowl, and drizzle with the fat. Add the sea salt, pepper, thyme, and garlic. Using a large spoon, gently toss to coat. In a round, well-greased baking dish, place the vegetable slices in a repeating pattern of concentric circles. You can also use a rectangular dish, and make a pattern of alternating rows. Add a bit more ghee on top of the vegetables, and cover with foil. Cook for 20 minutes, remove the foil, and baste the vegetables with the juices in the bottom of the pan. Cook for an additional 20 minutes, basting once again halfway through. Remove from the oven and serve.

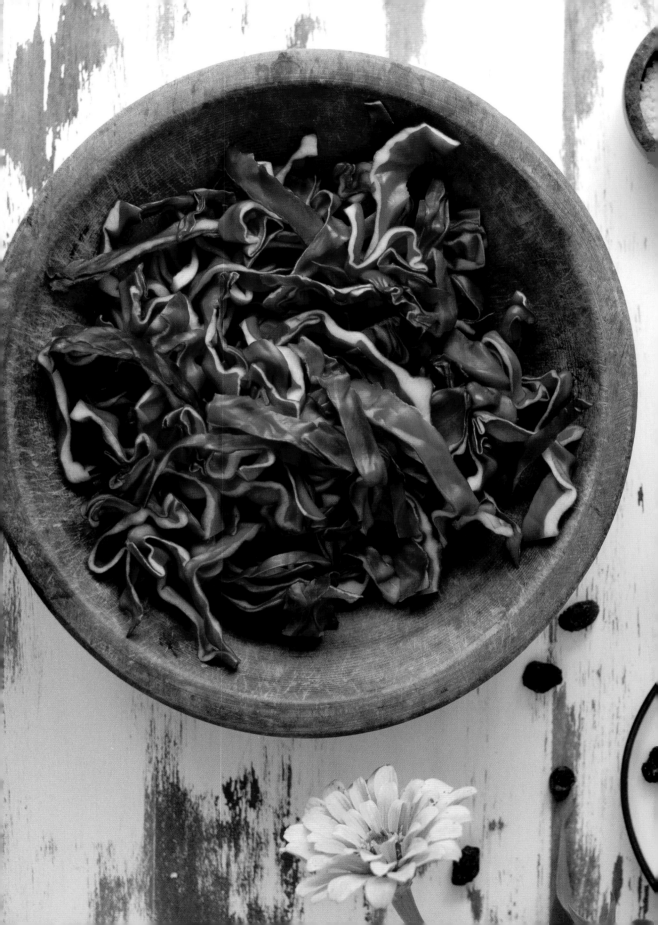

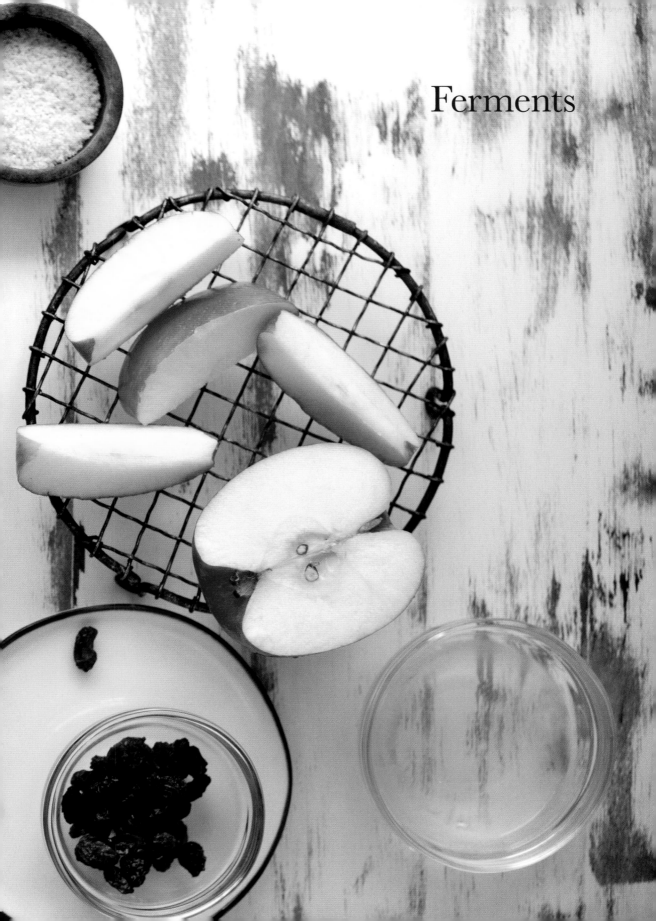

Ferments

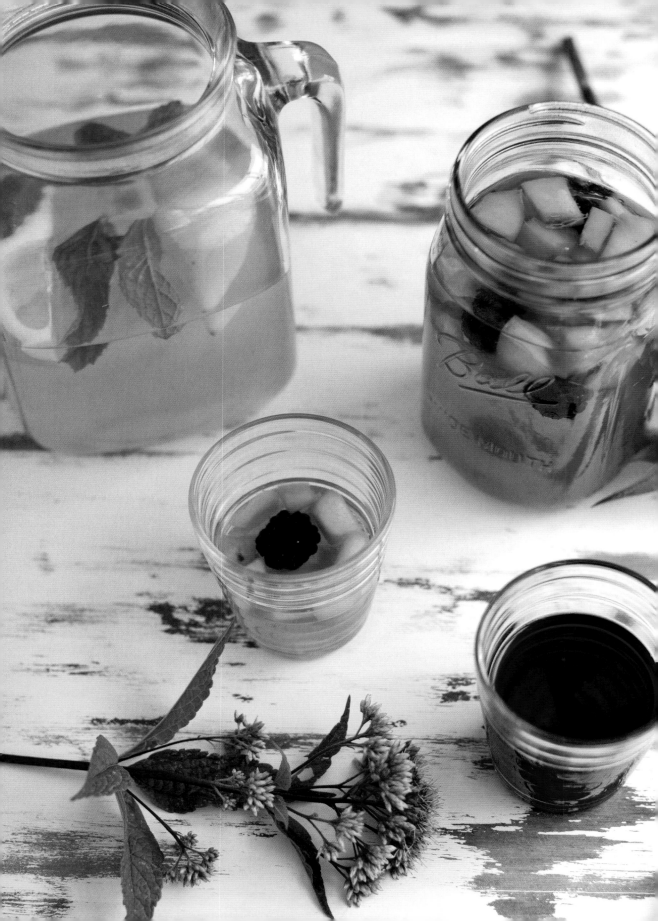

BEET KVASS
Makes 1 quart

Here's what Sally Fallon Morell says in *Nourishing Traditions* about Beet Kvass:

> This drink is valuable for its medicinal qualities and as a digestive aid. Beets are just loaded with nutrients. One 4-ounce glass, morning and night, is an excellent blood tonic, cleanses the liver, and is a good treatment for kidney stones and other ailments.

3 medium or 2 large organic beets, peeled and coarsely chopped
1 tablespoon sea salt
¼ cup whey or fermented pickle juice
2 cloves garlic, smashed or minced (optional)
Filtered water

Place the beets in a clean 2-quart widemouthed glass mason jar; add the salt, whey, and garlic, and fill to the shoulder with filtered water. Cap and leave on the counter for 2 days. Once you have drunk almost the entire first batch, you can add more filtered water, cap, and leave on the counter for an additional 2 days. After this you must throw out the beets and start fresh. Save ¼ cup liquid from your previous batch to use as an inoculant instead of the whey. The easiest way I find is to pour what you wish to drink, replace it with filtered water, and return the jar to the fridge. Do this each time you drink some kvass. When the beets are "spent," throw them out and start a new batch.

FRUIT KVASS
Makes 1 quart

1 cup organic fruit (fresh or frozen)
1-inch fresh ginger, peeled (optional, but
   I usually add to my ferments as it is so
   good for digestion)
Filtered water
Pinch of sea salt
½ cup whey

Place the fruit and ginger in a quart-sized mason jar, filling it about a quarter of the way up. Add filtered water up to the jar's shoulder, along with a pinch of sea salt and whey. Cap the jar tightly and leave it on the counter, at room temperature, for 2 to 3 days or until the lid is taut. Turn it upside down a few times a day. This is an anaerobic process, so be sure to keep the lid closed.

Depending on the temperature, your kvass may take a bit longer to ferment. You will see little bubbles starting to form; that means it's fermenting and the pressure is building in your jar. Be sure to check the lid to see if you can press it down or not. If you can't, that usually means the kvass is fermented and ready to drink.

You can strain out the fruit, if you wish, or enjoy it in your drink. This is a great way for our daughter to get a bit more fruit into her diet—following the fermentation process, the fruit's sugar content is largely or completely gone. The kvass will last in the fridge for about 1 week.

You can also use the same process as the beet kvass, above. Simply replace the amount of kvass you drink with water, every time, until the fruit becomes colorless and flavorless.

WATER KEFIR
Makes 1 quart

My kids love this beverage, and I am happy to give it to them, knowing that I am populating their little guts with yet more probiotics. Water kefir grains are available online (see resources); you can also ask for them at your local health food store. If you want sparkling kefir water, you have to invest in a Grolsch bottle to allow for more carbonation (see resources).

¼ cup organic sugar (coconut sugar is great if you have it)
1 quart filtered water, divided
Water kefir grains

Place the sugar in the bottom of a quart-sized mason jar and add ½ cup of hot filtered water. Give it a gentle stir to dissolve the sugar. Once the sugar is dissolved, add the remaining (cool) filtered water, leaving 2 to 4 inches at the top. Making sure that the water is cool, add the kefir grains, and gently stir again with a wooden spoon.

Cover the mason jar with some cloth and a rubber band, and let it sit on the counter for 24 to 48 hours. Once you have fermented the water, strain and drink as is; you can also do a second ferment by straining, adding to the jar ¼ cup fresh berries (or any of the ingredient combinations below), and leaving it to sit, covered for another day on the counter. This will add nice flavor and color to the water kefir. Cap, refrigerate, and start another batch.

Other kvass and water kefir combinations:

- Cherry, raspberry, cardamom
- Apple, ginger, raspberry
- Blueberry, lemon, mint
- Apple, raisins, cinnamon
- Lemon, dried apricots or prunes, ginger
- Mango, vanilla, chai spices
- Ginger, apple, lime
- Peach, chamomile, lemon
- Blackberry, peaches, vanilla bean
- Fresh lemon or lime
- 1 teaspoon Homemade Vanilla Extract (page 96)
- Mint, lime, ginger

LACTO-FERMENTED CILANTRO SALSA
Makes 1 quart

Many thanks to *Nourishing Traditions* for this delicious, money-saving recipe. You can make a quart of salsa for pennies, especially if you grow your own tomatoes! You can also switch out tomatoes with peaches if you like.

3 pounds fresh tomatoes, chopped, or
   1 jar or can (28 ounces) organic whole
   peeled tomatoes, liquid drained off
1 small onion, diced
1–2 cloves garlic, diced
1 serrano chile or jalapeño pepper,
   coarsely chopped (seeds optional)
1 teaspoon sea salt
1 teaspoon dried oregano
1 teaspoon ground coriander
1 teaspoon ground cumin
Cracked black pepper to taste
Juice of 1 lemon
Juice of 1 lime
½ cup whey or sauerkraut juice (I like
   Bubbie's sauerkraut juice or pickle juice,
   or I use my own if I have it on hand)
1 large bunch fresh cilantro, coarsely
   chopped

Place all of the ingredients (except the cilantro) in a food processor, and process until smooth and chunky. Add the cilantro, and pulse a few times. Place in a quart-sized, wide-mouthed mason jar, filling the jar up to its shoulder. Add filtered water if needed. Cover tightly, and keep at room temperature for about 3 days before transferring to the fridge. This will continue to ferment in the fridge and should be good for at least 4 to 6 weeks (peaches will be good for up to 4 weeks).

GINGER CARROTS
Makes 1 quart

Several years ago at a Weston A. Price conference, I had the pleasure of hearing Scott Grzybek of Zukay Live Foods speak about fermentation. His delightful demonstration on how to make ginger carrots was revelatory, as I had been spending a small fortune on them at the natural food store (no joke)! They are one of my absolute favorite ferments: delicious as a snack for kids and beautiful on a crudité platter for guests. This recipe can be used with broccoli and cauliflower as well.

4–6 carrots, peeled and cut into matchsticks
2-inch piece of ginger or 2 cloves garlic, sliced very thin
2 teaspoons sea salt
Starter culture (2 tablespoons whey, juice from previous batch, or vegetable starter culture from Cultures for Health; see resources)
Filtered water

In a bowl, thoroughly mix the carrot sticks, ginger, salt, and starter culture. Place in a quart-sized mason jar, and fill with filtered water to the shoulder, about 1 inch from the top. Shake the jar a bit and make sure that the culture and salt are evenly distributed. Place on your counter, out of the sun, for 2 to 4 weeks. Store in the fridge.

RED CABBAGE, RAISIN, AND APPLE SAUERKRAUT
Makes 1 quart

Monica Corrado, of Simply Being Well, introduced me to this easy and delicious sauerkraut recipe. It's my go-to kraut.

1 head red cabbage, cored and shredded
1 tablespoon sea salt
Handful of organic raisins
½ apple, grated
¼ cup whey (if not available, use an
   additional 1 tablespoon sea salt)
Filtered water

Thinly slice the cabbage with a knife, a mandoline, or the slicing blade of a food processor. Put the shredded cabbage in a large bowl with the salt, and massage until the juices are released (about 10 minutes). Add the raisins and grated apple, mix until well combined, then stuff in a widemouthed mason jar. The top of the cabbage should be at least 1 inch below the top of the jar. Be sure all the vegetables are covered with liquid. Add filtered water to cover. I usually tuck an extra cabbage leaf on top to make sure all the vegetables are submerged. Cover tightly, and keep at room temperature for about 3 days before transferring to cold storage. You can eat this sauerkraut immediately, but it improves with age.

FERMENTED FIG JAM
Makes 2 pints

This is a sweet treat. My kids love a little Fermented Fig Jam on a piece of Coconut Butter Bread (page 118), or with sliced apples and a nice raw cheese. It's also delicious with yogurt or kefir cheese and some homemade crackers. It will surely impress any guest! This was inspired by a blog called *Everyday Healthy Everyday Delicious*.

2 cups dried figs (I use a mix of Mission and Calimyrna)
1 cup hot filtered water
2 tablespoons raw honey
½ teaspoon sea salt
2 tablespoons whey or culture starter

Remove the stems from the figs. Place the figs in a bowl with the hot water, and let them soak for 15 minutes. (I've made this without soaking, too, but it makes for an easier blend if they're moist.) Place the figs along with their soaking water in a food processor and process until smooth. Add the honey, salt, and whey, and process to incorporate. Fill two pint-sized mason jars to the shoulder with the jam and cap. Leave on the counter for 2 to 3 days to ferment, then store in the fridge.

LACTO-FERMENTED JALAPEÑO HOT SLAW
Makes 1 quart

This recipe is inspired by Fab Ferments' Holy Jalapeno. I wish I had their secret recipe!

½ white cabbage, shredded

¼ Napa cabbage, shredded

2 tablespoons sea salt or 1 tablespoon
   sea salt plus ¼ cup whey

1 red onion, thinly sliced

2 jalapeños

1 bunch cilantro, chopped

5 radishes, sliced

½ teaspoon dried crushed chipotle chile

½ teaspoon dried crushed jalapeño chile

Place the cabbage in a large bowl. Add the salt, and massage for 3 to 5 minutes, until the juices release. You can also cover the bowl with a towel and leave it on the counter for 1 hour; the juices will release more. Add the remaining ingredients, and toss together (including the whey, if you are using it). With well-washed hands, stuff the cabbage mixture into a quart-sized glass mason jar, and push down with your fist to force the liquid to the top. You want the vegetables to be covered by liquid up to the shoulder (leaving 1 inch at the top). Cap and leave on the counter for 2 to 3 days. You can test the fermentation by pushing down on the lid to see if it clicks or not. If it does not click, it means the pressure has built up, and fermentation is happening.

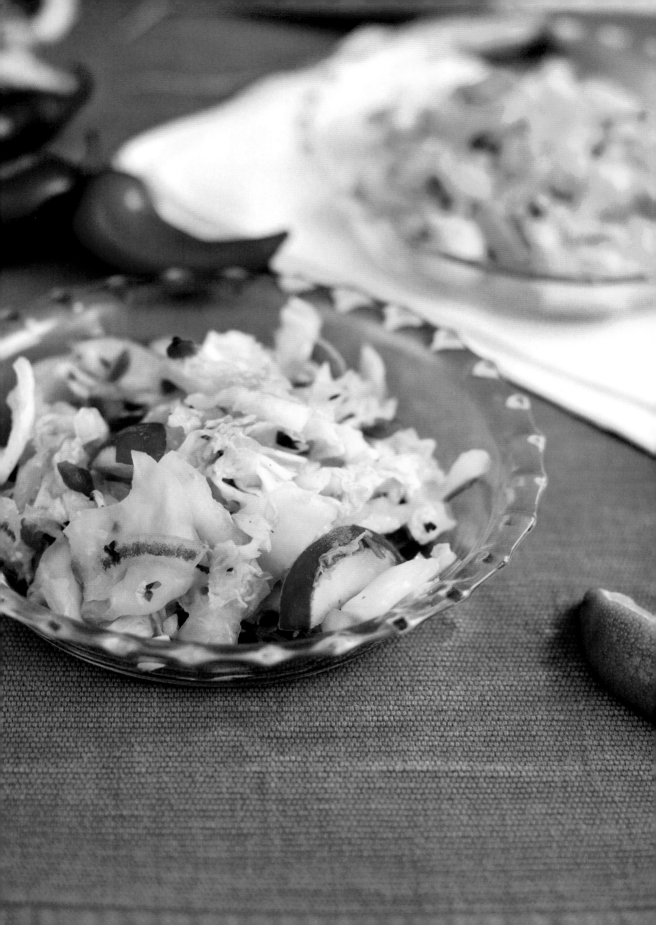

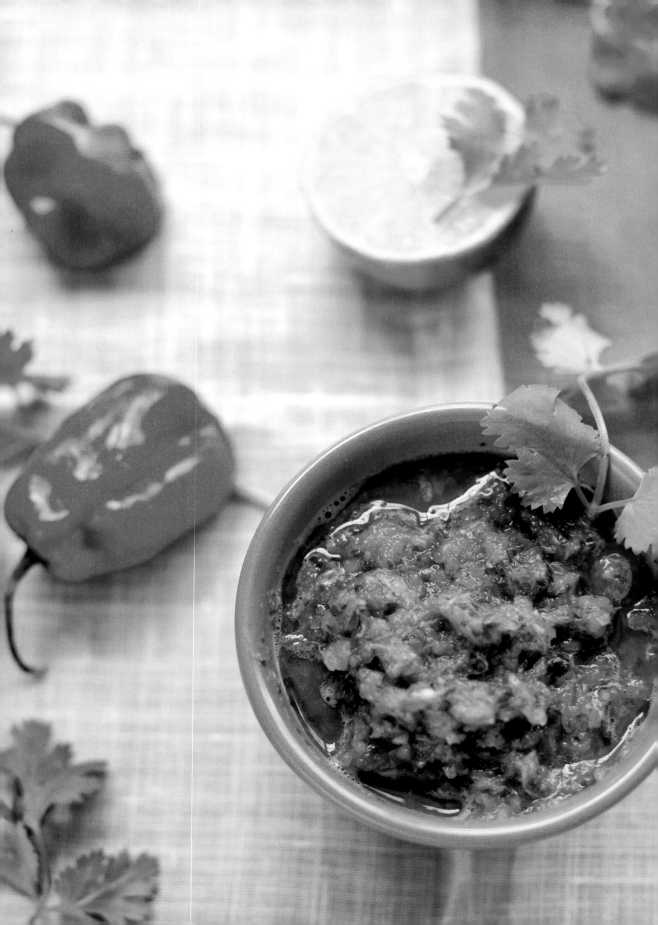

HOT NICKY
Makes 2 to 3 pint-sized mason jars

The Fabulous Fermented Hot Sauce!

Kerese, our dear friend from Trinidad, was with us in Maine a few summers back. We were making Mexican for dinner, and I grabbed my keys to hit the market and buy some hot sauce. She said, "Why don't we just make our own?" She then came along with me to the grocery, where I watched her put ten habanero peppers in the bag! We have been hooked on her amazing recipe ever since. In fact, for Nick's fortieth birthday we had a Mexican fiesta, and I gave away little pints of what we now call "Hot Nicky." Hot Nicky is great with any Mexican dish, or on burgers, eggs—you name it. But be careful, because you don't need much—just a teaspoon on the side, unless you're really daring. It's also delicious mixed with homemade mayo (page 107) on roast beef or fish, or as a yummy topping to oysters on the half shell.

¼ cup filtered water
½ lime, peeled
¾ bunch parsley
½ bunch scallions
1 onion
4–5 cloves garlic
5–10 habanero peppers (little orange
    hot peppers)
½ bunch cilantro
1–2 apples, peeled and cored (I often
    don't peel)
1 mango, peeled (optional)
Vegetable starter culture dissolved in ¼
    cup filtered water, or ¼ cup fresh whey
    or sauerkraut juice
Big pinch of sea salt

Mix all of the ingredients in a Vitamix or blender, using a tamper to help (if you're using a Vitamix). Store in pint-sized mason jars. Leave on the counter for 5 to 7 days. Store in the fridge.

LACTO-FERMENTED CURRY CAULIFLOWER KRAUT
Makes 1 quart

½ head Napa cabbage
½ head cauliflower, cut into small florets
1 tablespoon sea salt
1 bunch green onions, chopped
4 carrots, peeled and diced
1 white onion, thinly sliced
2 tablespoons curry
⅛ cup raisins (optional)

Add the cabbage and cauliflower to a bowl, and sprinkle with the salt. Massage the cabbage with your hands for 3 to 5 minutes, until it has released its juices. Add the remaining ingredients, and toss together. Follow the instructions above.

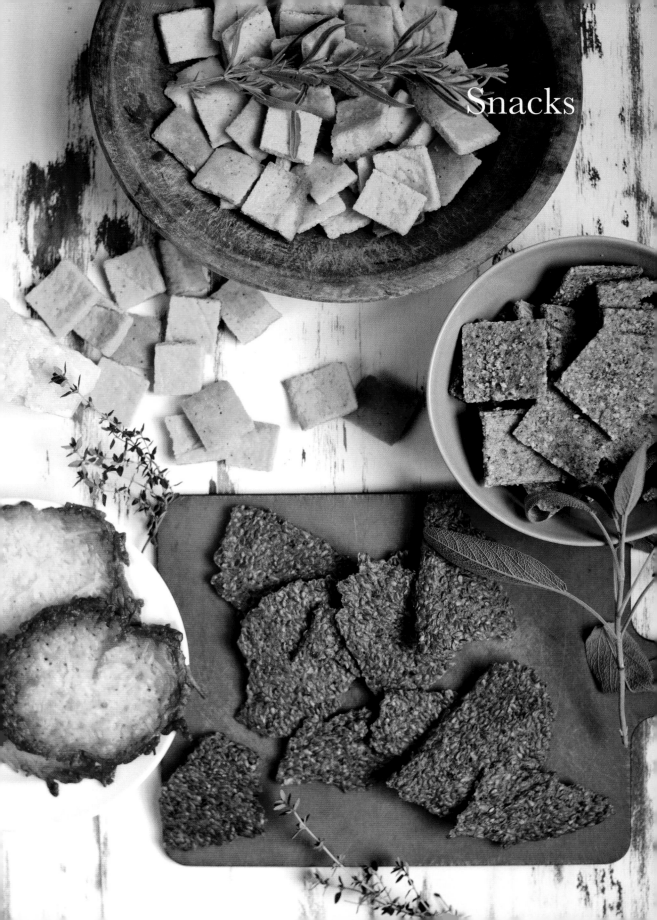

"CHEEZ-IT" KNOCKOFFS
Serves 6 to 8

This summer I saw my kids' eyes just watching their friends walking around with boxes of Cheez-Its. I decided to try creating a knockoff, and these became a perfect substitute!

1 cup coconut flour
¼ teaspoon sea salt
¼ teaspoon cayenne
¼ teaspoon white pepper
¼ teaspoon dried turmeric
¼ teaspoon garlic powder
3 cups shredded sharp cheddar cheese
1 cup shredded Parmesan
2 eggs
¼ cup grass-fed butter, softened

Preheat the oven to 350°F. Mix all the dry ingredients in a food processor and slowly add the cheese, eggs, and butter. When you can form the dough into a ball, roll it out between two pieces of parchment paper, or line a cookie sheet with parchment paper and press the dough evenly across the pan. Bake the crackers for 10 minutes. At this point you can gently cut them into little squares the size of Cheez-Its. Place the crackers back in the oven for an additional 10 minutes. Remove the crackers, and break them up into squares. Once they're all broken up, put them back into a turned-off oven or the dehydrator to crisp up. Watch carefully in the oven, as they will burn quickly. Once they're cool, these crackers can be stored in an airtight container—although these don't last long in my house.

SWEET CRACKERS
Makes 30 to 40 crackers

These are great with cultured cream (page 30) into which you've folded honey and cinnamon.

2 cups almond flour

½ teaspoon sea salt

1 tablespoon cinnamon

2 tablespoons cacao powder

1 teaspoon Homemade Vanilla Extract
  (page 96)

1 egg or chia egg replacer
  (see note below)

1 teaspoon alcohol-free chocolate extract
  (optional)

1–2 tablespoons coconut oil

In a food processor or mixing bowl, add all of the dry ingredients; gradually add in the wet until you can form a ball with your dough. Pop this into the fridge for about 20 minutes. Roll out the dough between two pieces of parchment paper. This will help keep it from sticking to your rolling pin. Once the dough is about ⅛ inch thick, score it with your knife in nice cracker shapes. Place them gently on a nonstick sheet in your dehydrator, and dehydrate at 145°F for 12 hours. Flip the crackers, and dehydrate for another 12 hours. Store in an airtight container in the fridge to keep fresh.

If you don't have a dehydrator, place the crackers on a parchment-lined cookie sheet in the oven at its lowest temperature for about an hour, flipping halfway through. Watch them to see when they crisp, as every oven is different. They will crisp up more as they cool down.

Note: *To make a chia egg, combine 1 tablespoon of ground chia seeds with 3 tablespoons of filtered water, and let stand for 5 minutes.*

ONION CRACKERS / BREAD
Serves 8 to 10

3 large sweet yellow onions
¾ cup raw sunflower seeds, finely
   ground into meal with a food processor
   (be careful not to make nut butter)
½ cup coconut aminos
½ teaspoon sea salt
1 carrot, shredded
1 zucchini, shredded
⅓ cup olive oil
1 cup ground flax seeds
Sesame, poppy, and/or pumpkin seeds,
   to garnish the top

In a food processor, mix the onions, sunflower seed meal, coconut aminos, salt, carrot, zucchini, and olive oil until smooth. Add the flax seeds, and blend until well incorporated. Spread thinly on nonstick sheets, and sprinkle with a variety of seeds for garnish. Be sure to press these into the batter gently with the back of a fork, so they stick once the crackers have been dehydrated. Dehydrate at 110°F for 6 hours. Carefully flip the crackers, and dehydrate for another couple of hours. Cut or break crackers into your desired sizes. Put them back into the dehydrator, and dehydrate for an additional 18 to 24 hours. Store in airtight containers in the fridge. You may want to double the batch, as these will get gobbled up quickly!

Note: *If you want to take it up a notch, you can caramelize your onions first! Slice and cook for 30 minutes with a pinch of sea salt and 2 tablespoons of coconut oil or ghee in a large sauté pan over medium-low heat.*

PARMESAN CRISPS
Serves 6

This is an awesome gluten-free cracker option!

1½ cups shredded Parmesan

Preheat the oven to 350°F. Place a piece of parchment paper on a baking sheet. Evenly space 6 (¼-cup) mounds of Parmesan cheese on the paper. Gently pat down each mound to flatten it into a round 4½ to 5 inches in diameter. Bake for 8 to 10 minutes, until golden and bubbly. Remove from the oven and let cool.

These keep for a while stored in a ziplock bag in the fridge. Heat them in the toaster oven, or enjoy them at room temperature. They're even delicious cold!

SIMPLE FLAX CRACKERS
Makes 20 to 30 crackers

I discovered flax crackers one day in the grocery store, and after spending $40 on crackers, in various flavors, that were all gone in about 2 days in my house I decided I could knock these suckers off. You can get creative and add a blend of Mexican spices, Italian seasonings, or even cinnamon and pumpkin pie spice for sweet crackers.

4 cups flax seeds
2 cups pumpkin or sunflower seeds,
   soaked (see page 19 for soaking chart)
1 tablespoon sea salt
5 tablespoons coconut aminos (optional)
1 bunch fresh cilantro
1 bunch fresh parsley
Zest and juice of 1 lime
1 teaspoon black pepper

Put the flax seeds in a bowl, and cover with filtered water. Let them soak for 6 hours. Add all of the ingredients, except the flax, to your food processor. Blend until you reach a slightly chunky consistency. Add the flax, and blend until well incorporated. The flax will not be ground. Spread the dough out on three nonstick dehydrator sheets, and dehydrate at 90°F for 10 to 12 hours. At this point, flip the giant cracker (you can score it into desired cracker shapes if you wish—we just break it up at the end) onto a standard drying sheet, and dehydrate for another 10 to 12 hours or until crisp. This will allow it to cook evenly on both sides. Break up into smaller crackers and enjoy.

Variations: Get creative, and add spices for your own yummy creation. Try sprinkling with 1 to 2 tablespoons Taco Seasoning (page 128) once you have spread the cracker on the dehydrator sheet, or mix 3 tablespoons Taco Seasoning right into the batter.

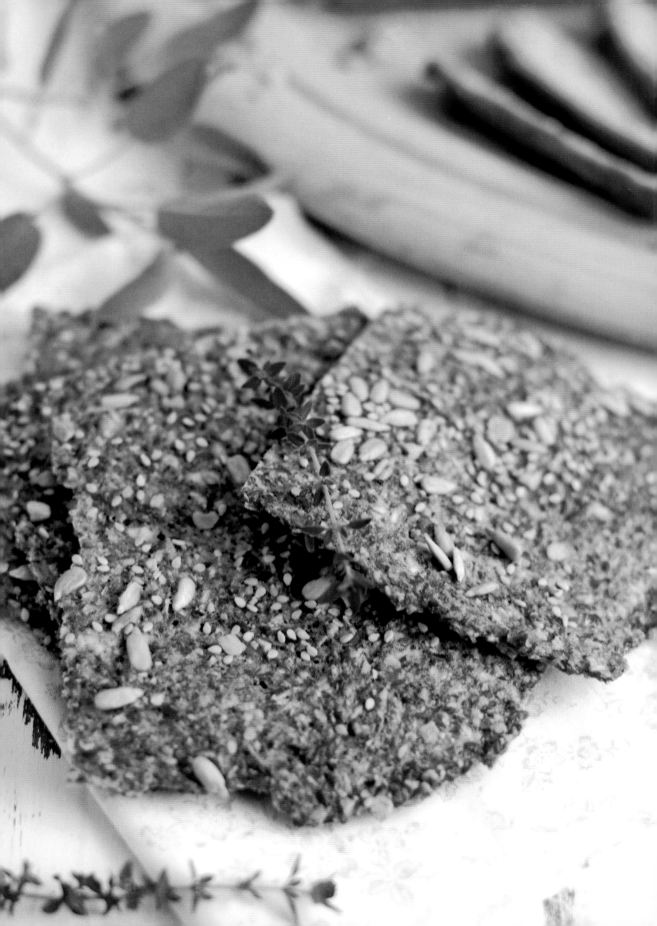

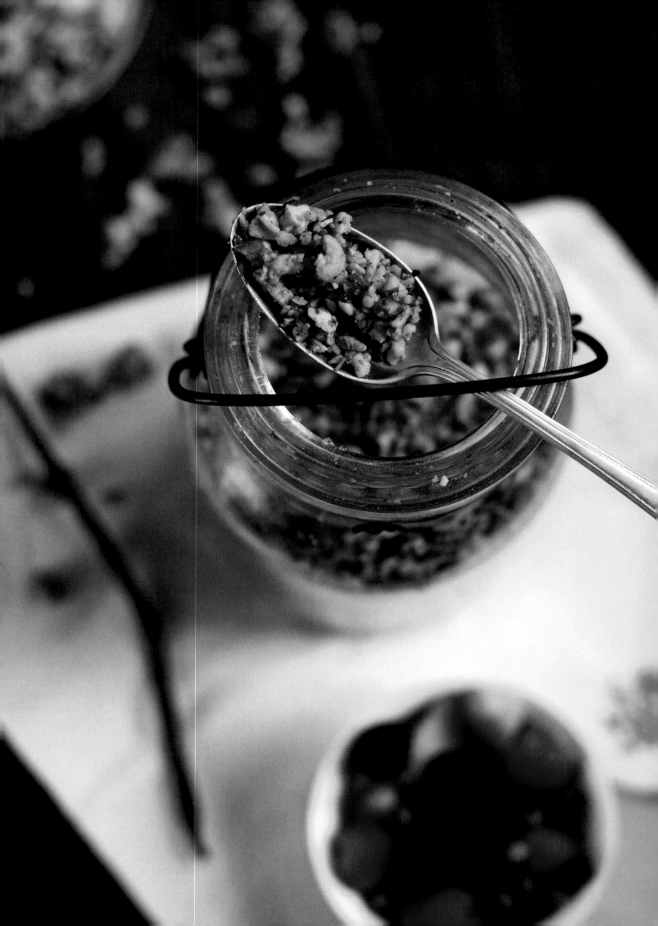

GRANOLA THREE WAYS

Granola is a great treat for our family. I don't make it all the time, because it's expensive and disappears too quickly in our house. But it's a nice alternative to eggs, meats, and soups for breakfast once in a while! It also makes a healthy snack on the go. We enjoy it with homemade nut milk (page 19), homemade coconut milk (page 23), or as a topping to homemade kefir (page 28) or yogurt (page 27)

Granola #1
Makes 1 quart

3 cups whichever nuts and seeds you wish, soaked (see page 19 for soaking chart)

¼ cup coconut oil

½ teaspoon sea salt

1–2 tablespoons vanilla (page 96) or almond extract

2 teaspoons cinnamon

Scrapings of 1 vanilla bean

1 chia egg (see note below)

1 cup applesauce (I like homemade with skins on, but don't sweat it if it comes from a jar)

½ cup shredded coconut (optional)

Note: *To make a chia egg, combine 1 tablespoon of ground chia seeds with 3 tablespoons of filtered water and let stand for 5 minutes.*

Granola #2
Makes 1 quart

2 cups nuts, soaked

1 cup seeds, soaked

½ cup dried apples, chopped

5 dried figs, chopped

2 teaspoons cinnamon

½ teaspoon sea salt

2 tablespoons vanilla extract (page 96)

¼ cup coconut oil

½ cup shredded coconut (optional)

Granola #3
Makes 1 quart

½ cup cashews, soaked
½ cup pecans, soaked
½ cup sunflower seeds, soaked
½ cup pumpkin seeds, soaked
2 tablespoons cinnamon
1 teaspoon vanilla extract
½ teaspoon nutmeg
½ teaspoon sea salt
½ cup pumpkin puree
½ cup shredded coconut (optional)
¼ cup coconut oil

Pulse all of the ingredients together in a food processor until a very chunky paste is formed. Spread on your dehydrator's nonstick drying sheet and set at 145°F for 12 to 24 hours, stirring once or twice. (Or spread on a cookie sheet and bake in the oven on its lowest possible setting for 12 to 24 hours, depending on temperature.) Break up the granola; store in an airtight container in the fridge.

TOASTED COCONUT CHIP TRAIL MIX
Serves 4 to 6

2 cups large coconut chips
2 tablespoons coconut oil
1 teaspoon cinnamon
½ cup nuts of choice
½ cup dried fruit
Pinch of sea salt
Cocoa nibs (optional)

Place the coconut chips in a skillet, and add the coconut oil. Heat on low, tossing to coat. Once the chips are slightly golden, remove them from the heat, place them in a bowl, and add the cinnamon. Toss to coat. Once they're cool, add the remaining ingredients and toss. Store in an airtight container in the fridge. This is a great on-the-go snack or for school lunches. An even easier coconut snack is to place coconut in a skillet, or toaster oven, with 2 heaping tablespoons coconut oil and a pinch of salt. Heat until golden. This is a good popcorn replacement for those who love coconut. Careful—it is addicting!

CRISPY KALE CHIPS
Serves 6 to 8

1 head kale (I like the flat lacinato kale or
   curly kale)
1 tablespoon coconut aminos
1–2 tablespoons coconut oil
1½ cups large coconut flakes

Preheat the oven to 350°F. Rip the kale leaves into bite-sized pieces, discarding the heavy stalks. Spread the kale evenly across a baking sheet. Drizzle with the coconut aminos, and add dollops of coconut oil. Top with shredded coconut.

Place in the oven, and toss after 1 to 2 minutes once the coconut oil has melted. Bake for 10 to 12 minutes, until the coconut is deeply golden brown, tossing two or three times along the way. Turn off the oven, and let the kale sit inside to crisp up any remaining soft pieces (about 10 minutes, watching carefully so as not to burn). Remove from the oven and serve. This is a great snack and will stay fresh in an airtight container in the fridge.

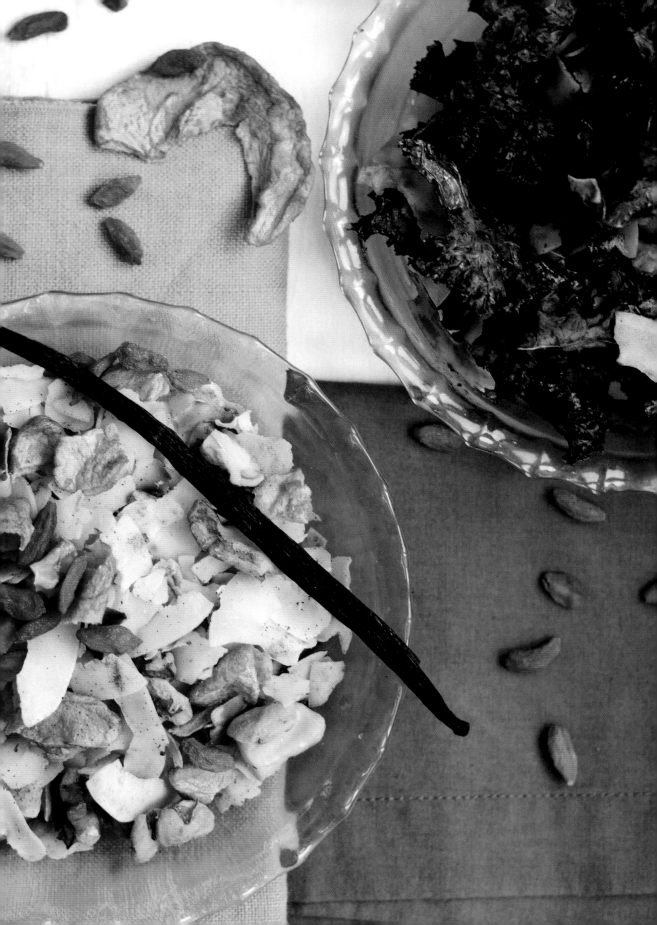

COCONUT CURRY HAZELNUTS
Serves 4 to 6

These are another expensive grocery store treat that I knocked off!

2 tablespoons raw honey
1 cup hazelnuts
½ cup finely shredded coconut
1 teaspoon curry powder
Pinch of sea salt

Very lightly melt the honey so as to not destroy the enzymes. Mix all of the ingredients together, and place on a parchment-lined cookie sheet in the refrigerator to solidify. Cut into squares; store in the fridge. Enjoy!

NUT PULP

Nut pulp is what you have left after making nut milk (page 19). It's a wonderful ingredient, so don't throw it away. There are so many ways to use it; I could have included ten more recipes for you to try! Here are a few favorites to get you started.

Chocolate Truffles
Makes 12 to 15 truffles

1¼ cups nut pulp, coconut pulp, or almond meal
¼ cup honey
1 teaspoon cinnamon
1 teaspoon vanilla extract (page 96), or scrapings of 2 vanilla beans
Generous pinch of sea salt
1 cup dried shredded coconut
¼ cup cacao powder with a little extra for rolling the truffles

Mix all of the ingredients together in a food processor, adding a little filtered water as needed if the dough is too dry. Place the dough in the fridge for about 10 minutes to allow the flavors to marry and to make it more workable. Remove from the fridge, and use a spoon to break off about 1-inch-diameter balls. Roll the balls between your palms, then roll in extra cacao powder and place on a plate. Store in the fridge.

Macaroons
Makes 12 to 15 cookies

1 cup nut pulp or coconut pulp
¼ cup honey or 6 Medjool dates, pitted
1½ cups dried coconut flakes
3 tablespoons coconut oil
1 tablespoon vanilla extract (page 96) or scrapings of 2 vanilla beans
Pinch of sea salt

Place all of the ingredients in a food processor, and process until a dough forms. Place in the fridge for about 10 minutes to allow the flavors to marry and to make the dough more workable. Remove from the fridge, and use a spoon to break off 1-inch-diameter balls. Roll the balls between your palms, place on your dehydrating tray, and press down to flatten to more of a cookie shape. Dehydrate at 115°F for 4 to 6 hours. If you're short on time, leave as balls, place on cookie sheet and pop in the fridge to chill.

Gingersnaps
Makes 12 to 15 cookies

1 cup nut pulp or coconut pulp
1½ cups shredded coconut
6 dates
¼ teaspoon ground nutmeg
¼ teaspoon ground ginger
Pinch of allspice
½ teaspoon cinnamon
1 teaspoon vanilla extract (page 96), or
   scrapings of 2 vanilla beans

Mix all of the ingredients together in a food processor. Place in the fridge for about 10 minutes to let the flavors marry and to make the dough more workable. Remove from the fridge, and use a spoon to break off 1-inch-diameter balls. Roll the balls between your palms and eat as is, or place on your dehydrating tray, and press down to flatten to more of a cookie shape. Dehydrate at 115°F for 4 to 6 hours. If you do not have a dehydrator, place the cookies in your oven on the lowest possible setting and bake for 1 to 2 hours or until they achieve your desired crispness. Store in the fridge.

Nut Pulp Hummus
Makes 1 to 2 cups

This is a great alternative to chickpeas. My children did not know the difference! They use it as a dip for raw vegetables.

1–2 cups nut pulp
3 cloves garlic
Juice of 1 lemon
6 tablespoons raw tahini
2 teaspoons ground cumin
Pinch of cayenne
Sea salt and pepper
1 tablespoon olive oil,
   plus more for garnish
1 tablespoon red palm oil (optional but
   adds a nice color and different fatty
   acid profile)
Sprinkle of paprika, for garnish

Place all of the ingredients in a food processor, and blend for 1 minute or until smooth. Remove to a bowl, and drizzle with olive oil and a sprinkle of paprika.

Nut Pulp "Cheese Spread"
Makes 1 to 2 cups

1–2 cups nut pulp
¼ cup olive oil
Juice of 1 lemon
¼ cup chopped fresh herbs
2 cloves garlic, pressed
½ cup diced onion
½ teaspoon sea salt
Fresh cracked pepper

Mix all of the ingredients together in a food processor to your desired consistency, and serve with vegetables or Nut Crackers (page 21).

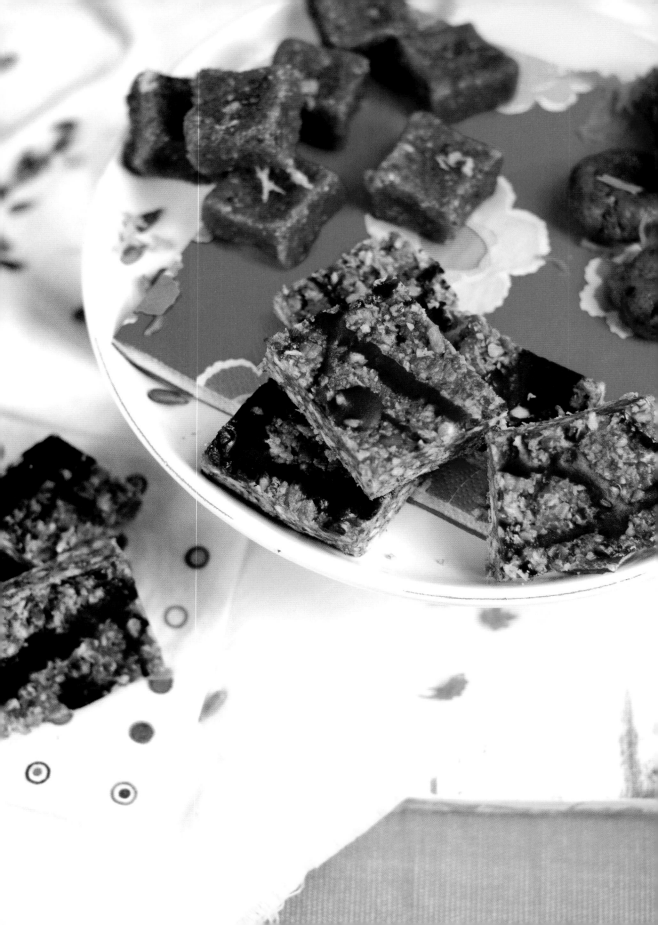

NATURAL NUTTY "ENERGY BARS"
Serves 15 to 20

Back in my days of fat-free living, I thought it was healthy to survive on energy bars filled with soy protein isolate and other laboratory ingredients. In fact, I used to be a rep for one of the companies handing out free samples at cool ski events, mountain bike races, or marathons, so unfortunately, I had an endless free supply. They became my lunch for about two years . . . dreadful to even think! Of course, I learned my lesson: You should never subsist on processed foods at the risk of your health and wellness. This recipe is a healthy variation on those weird engineered bars from long ago (which unfortunately are now all over grocery store shelves). It makes a delicious, nutrient-dense snack that I am happy to share with my kids: on the go, in their school lunches, or as an after-meal treat. Be mindful of going overboard with nuts, though, and limit the serving size to two small bars. "One for each hand," as my sister-in-law says. This recipe is inspired by Kayla at Radiant Life!

2½ cups sprouted nuts (use a variety, like walnuts, cashews, and pecans)
1½ cups sprouted seeds (use a variety, like sesame, sunflower, and pumpkin)
½ cup chia seeds (optional)
1 cup shredded unsweetened coconut or coconut flakes
1 teaspoon cinnamon (optional)
½ teaspoon sea salt, plus a pinch
½ cup coconut oil
¼–½ cup raw honey, or 6 dates, soaked and pureed
2 teaspoons vanilla extract
Homemade Chocolate Sauce (page 271) or "Nutella" (recipe follows) (optional, if tolerated)

Place the nuts, seeds, chia, shredded coconut, cinnamon, and ½ teaspoon sea salt in a food processor, and pulse to a coarse consistency. Depending on your preference, you can also process more finely. Place a saucepan over medium-low heat, and lightly melt the coconut oil. Turn off the heat, and add the honey (or dates), pinch of salt, and vanilla to incorporate. Add the shredded coconut mixture to the pot, and fold to incorporate. Place in a parchment-lined or well-greased pan. Grease your hands with a little coconut oil, and press the mixture evenly throughout the pan. Drizzle with Chocolate Sauce or top with "Nutella," if you like. Cool in the fridge for 30 minutes to 1 hour. Cut into bars and serve.

"Nutella"
Makes about 2 cups

For all those worried about cocoa and its legality on the GAPS Diet, a friend of mine nicely pointed me to Dr. Natasha's site, www.gaps.me. There she states:

> Cocoa powder is permissible once digestive problems have subsided . . . I find that many people can start having it occasionally on the Full GAPS Diet, once the digestive symptoms are gone. Find pure organic cocoa powder. Mixing the powder with some honey and sour cream makes a delicious dessert, and you can add it to your homemade ice cream or cakes. After trying it for the first time, observe your patient for any reactions. Cocoa is very rich in magnesium and some essential amino acids and, unless your digestive system is not ready for it, there is no need to avoid.

2 cups soaked or crispy hazelnuts (page 18)
2 tablespoons raw cocoa powder
1 tablespoon raw honey
2–4 tablespoons melted coconut oil
Pinch of sea salt

Blend the nuts in a food processor until smooth, then add in the other ingredients. Process until uniformly incorporated.

HOMEMADE "LARA BARS"
Makes 8 to 10 small bars

Get creative with this recipe. You can use different nuts, or add in coconut shreds, cacao powder, or nibs. Try subbing apricots or prunes for the dates. Let your kids roll them in coconut!

¾ cup cashews (or nuts of choice)
¼ cup walnuts
5 pitted Medjool dates
Dash of cinnamon
Zest of 1 lemon
¼ teaspoon sea salt
½ teaspoons vanilla extract (page 96)
Handful of goji berries, golden berries, or dried blueberries (optional)

Process the nuts in a food processor until you reach a fine consistency. Add the remaining ingredients (except the berries). Pulse until combined. Add the berries in for some color and extra nutritional punch! Mold into squares or balls, and place in the fridge for 1 to 2 hours. You can also spread the mixture in a pan or roll out between two pieces of parchment, chill well, then cut into bars.

CARROT CAKE COOKIES
Makes 15 cookies

1 cup nut butter of choice
½ cup finely shredded coconut
2 teaspoons vanilla extract (page 96)
2 teaspoons cinnamon
⅛ teaspoon allspice
½ teaspoon sea salt
½ cup chopped dates
½ cup chopped walnuts or
  nuts of choice
1 finely shredded carrot

Mix all of the ingredients together by hand. Using a spoon, scoop out tablespoon-sized dollops, and roll into balls between your palms. Let the cookies set in the fridge, and store them in the fridge or freezer.

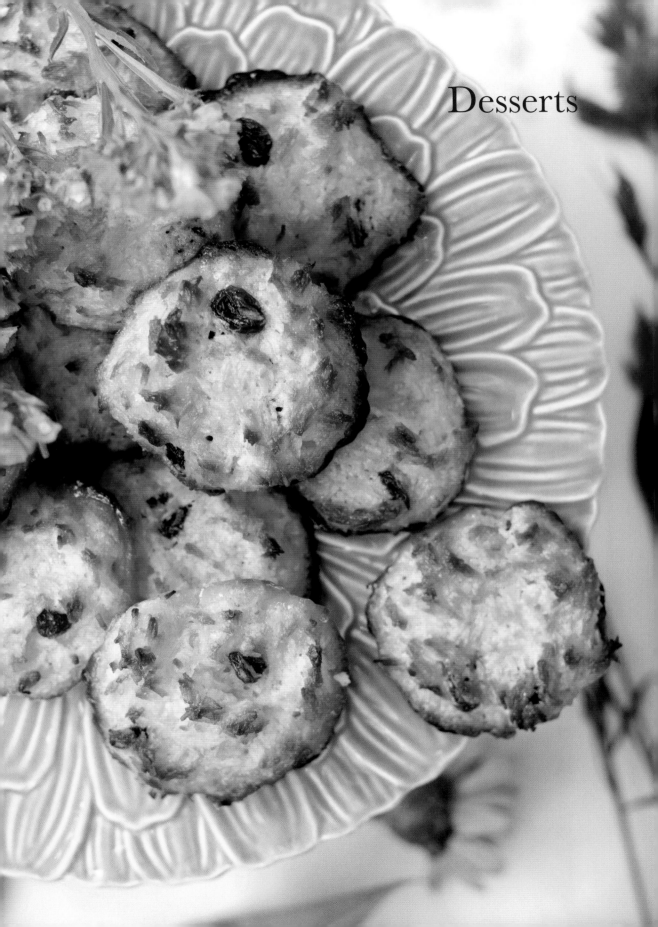

Desserts

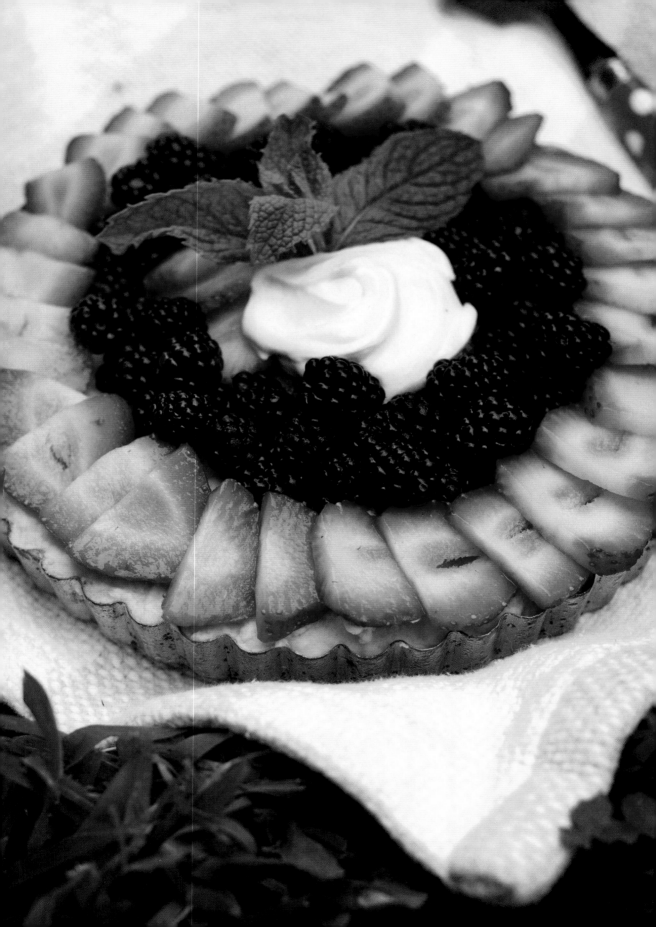

SUMMER BERRY TART WITH RAW NUT CRUST
Serves 6 to 8

All my life, I've admired the exquisite tarts displayed in gourmet bakeries and wondered how in the world they were made. Then I decided to just go ahead and try it myself. The trick is using beautiful fruit at the peak of freshness and a tart pan with fancy scalloped edges . . . instant gourmet!

Crust

1 cup soaked or crispy walnuts (page 18)
1 cup dried shredded coconut

1 pinch sea salt
5 dates

Filling

2 tablespoons raw honey
2 cups cultured cream

Pinch of sea salt

Fruit

Fresh, in-season berries of choice (blueberries, raspberries, blackberries, strawberries, cherries, boysenberries, elderberries, mulberries . . . shall I go on?)

Place all of the crust ingredients in your food processor, and process until a slightly rough paste is formed. Spread and press evenly into an 8-inch tart pan. Place in the fridge for 30 minutes to harden.

For the filling, ever so gently fold the honey into the cultured cream. Be careful not to whip it, as it will quickly turn to butter. Spread evenly on top of crust, and place in the fridge for another 30 minutes.

Select your fruit of choice, and have fun placing it on top in a decorative way. Add a sprig of mint and you are gourmet, baby!

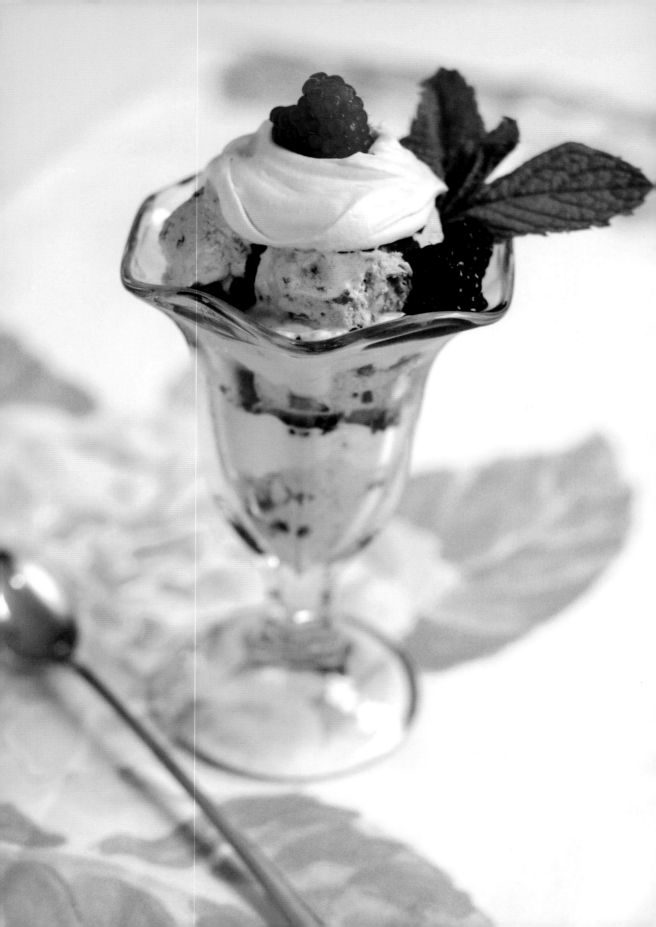

ICE CREAM

I have been experimenting with different dairy-free ice creams, and without egg yolks, the consistency has been either icy, or not hard enough. Adding yolks to your ice cream is also a great nutrition booster, so unless you're suffering from an egg allergy, add a few to each batch. It was also a good way for us to test egg yolk with our daughter. She's often refused trying egg in a smoothie or juice, but ice cream she'll never refuse! And it's a great way to get gelatin into your diet.

Here's a great tip: Make sure your ice cream maker insert has been in the freezer for at least 24 hours. In fact, get in the habit of storing it there if you have room, so that you are always prepared to make ice cream. I also store the coconut milk in the fridge, or at least place it in there for a few hours (or the freezer for 1 hour) before using.

Finally, being able to make our own ice cream really helped us through a long, hot summer in Maine with no trips to the Ice Cream Factory (a historically standard outing for the Boynton family). The kids were content to make their own treats, and they especially enjoyed helping to concoct flavors and taste test new recipes. Here are a few of our favorites.

Banana Nut Butter Ice Cream
Serves 8 to 10

4 very ripe bananas with spots, frozen
¼ cup nut butter
3 tablespoons raw honey
¼ cup coconut milk
1 tablespoon gelatin
1 teaspoon vanilla extract (page 96)
2 organic pastured egg yolks (optional)

Chop frozen bananas into 1-inch pieces, and add to the blender. Add the remaining ingredients, and blend until smooth. Start the ice cream maker, and slowly pour in the banana mixture. Process for about 20 minutes or until your desired consistency is achieved. At the end you can add some chopped unsweetened chocolate and chopped walnuts, if you'd like a chunky ice cream. Banana is very versatile, so feel free to leave out the nut butter and add other berries or a tablespoon of cinnamon, or eat as is!

Vanilla Chocolate Chip
Serves 8 to 10

2 cans full-fat coconut milk (Native Forest brand uses BPA-free cans and offers a version free of guar gum—which is not allowed on GAPS)

Scrapings of 4 vanilla beans

1 teaspoon vanilla extract (page 96)

¼ cup unsweetened chocolate shreds or cocoa nibs (if tolerated)

1 tablespoon gelatin

¾ cup raw honey

2 organic pastured egg yolks (optional)

Blend all of the ingredients in a blender. Turn on the ice cream maker, and slowly pour in the vanilla mixture. Process for 10 to 20 minutes, or until your desired consistency is reached. Remove to another container, and freeze. This is truly a yummy chocolate chip ice cream. Add some peppermint extract or fresh mint for a delicious mint chocolate chip!

Berry Ice Cream
Serves 8 to 10

I created this simple ice cream for our daughter, who just cannot do honey or banana. She seems to be fine with a little stevia here and there, so I was happy to be able to give her this ice cream. We had tried a few with honey, but her seizures did increase.

½ cup blackberries (or berries of choice)

½ cup raspberries (or berries of choice)

2 cans full-fat coconut milk (Native Forest brand uses BPA-free cans and offers a version free of guar gum—which is not allowed on GAPS)

1 tablespoon gelatin

2 teaspoons vanilla extract (page 96)

3 tablespoons raw honey (or 20 drops liquid stevia, or a few pinches of green powdered stevia)

2 organic pastured egg yolks (optional)

Mix half the berries in a blender with the coconut milk, gelatin, vanilla, honey, and egg yolks (if you're using them). This creates a beautiful pink ice cream. Fold in the remaining berries whole. Turn on the ice cream maker, and pour in slowly. Churn until frozen or desired consistency is reached, 10 to 20 minutes. Scoop out, and store in a separate container in the freezer.

CHOCOLATE SAUCE
Makes ½ cup

This will harden when put on top of cold ice cream. It is almost like a healthy version of Magic Shell. We don't typically add the honey, as the ice cream is sweet enough.

2–3 tablespoons coconut oil
1 bar unsweetened dark chocolate
Pinch of sea salt
1 tablespoon raw honey (optional)

Melt all of the ingredients together in a saucepan over low heat. Store in a glass container.

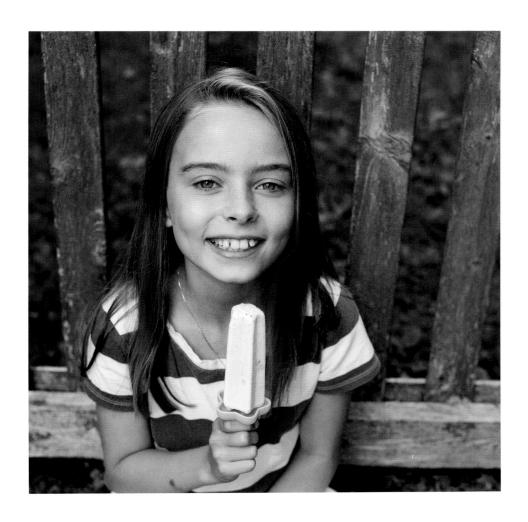

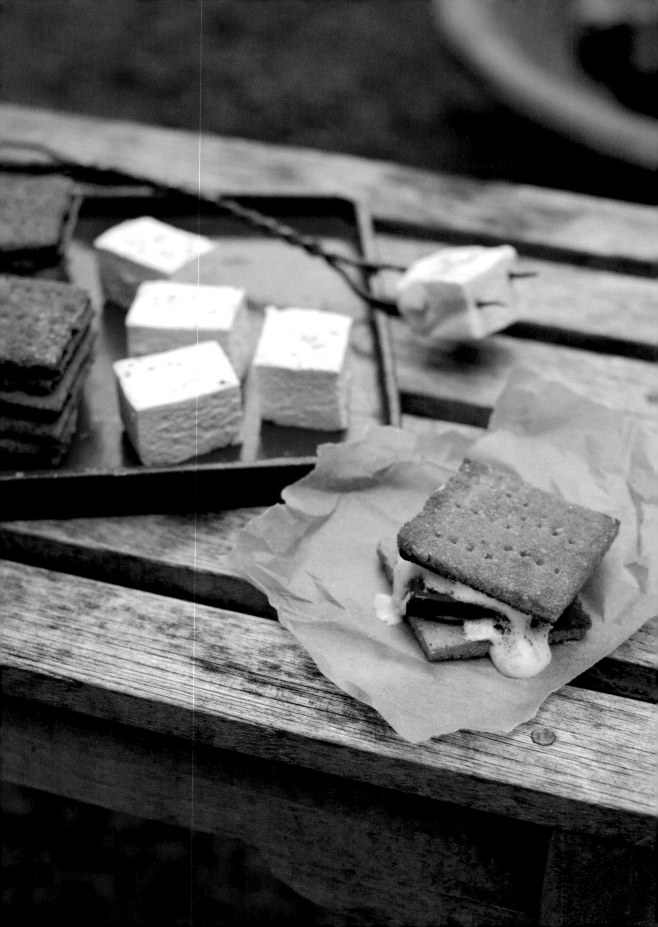

CAN YOU SAY S'MORES?
Makes 20 to 30 marshmallows

This saved the day when my triplets were at summer camp and wanted to make s'mores with their friends. What was I to do, make them yet another "different" treat? I just couldn't do it! This totally works, and it really doesn't take long at all! The cookbook *Internal Bliss* guided me through this delicious number.

3 tablespoons unflavored gelatin
1 cup ice-cold filtered water, divided
1 cup organic honey
1 teaspoon vanilla or other organic extract (page 96)
Scrapings of 1 vanilla bean
¼ teaspoon sea salt
Coconut oil or ghee, for greasing the top

Thoroughly grease an 8 by 8-inch pan and line with paper, bottom and sides. Leave some length to use as handles when you remove your finished marshmallows.

In the bowl of a standing mixer, soften and dissolve the gelatin with ½ cup of the water. Mix on low to incorporate. Meanwhile, pour the other ½ cup water into a saucepan along with the honey, vanilla, and salt. Bring the mixture to a gentle boil over medium-high heat. Place a candy thermometer in the saucepan and continue to boil, whisking periodically, until it reaches 240°F. It may seem to hover around 225°F for a while, but then suddenly will shoot to 240°F. This will take approximately 7 to 8 minutes. Remove the pan from the heat.

With your mixer on low, slowly pour the honey mixture into the bowl, combining it with the softened gelatin. Turn the mixer to high, and continue beating for about 10 minutes, until it becomes thick like marshmallow crème.

Turn off the mixer, and pour the marshmallow crème into the parchment-lined pan. Lightly grease your hands with coconut oil or ghee, and smooth out the top. This will keep the crème from sticking to your fingers. Let set on the counter for a few hours or overnight. When set, remove the marshmallows by lifting the parchment paper. Cut to your desired sizes. You will be amazed: These are just like store-bought marshmallows, without all the added junk! Enjoy with some unsweetened or honey-sweetened chocolate (if tolerated) and a few homemade Graham Crackers (recipe follows). Be careful when toasting these marshmallows. They do melt rather than crisping up.

Graham Crackers
Makes 20 to 30 crackers

4½ cups almond flour
1 teaspoon gelatin
2 teaspoons cinnamon (reserve 1 for sprinkling on top)
½ cup honey
1 teaspoon vanilla extract (page 96)
¼ cup coconut oil, butter, or lard

Preheat the oven to 350°F. Place all of the dry ingredients in a food processor, and blend until well incorporated. Add the wet ingredients, and blend again.

Grease a jelly-roll pan, line with parchment paper, and grease again.

Gently and evenly press the mixture onto the pan. It might seem like there isn't enough, but just keep working it around with your palm and fingertips until the pan is evenly filled. Using a knife, score the dough into rectangles and poke with a fork to make them look like traditional graham crackers. Bake for about 12 minutes. Let them cool and remove from the pan.

Depending on evenness of browning, you might want to turn the oven off, flip the crackers, and lightly bake the other side for an additional 1 to 2 minutes, watching carefully as not to burn.

COCONUT BARK

This is one of those recipes that you will try once and then start creating your own! Be sure to go to makenmold.com under the bark section to find a chocolate bar mold (see resources).

To soften the coconut butter, place the jar in a pot of water covering ¾ of the way up the side of the jar. Bring the water to a boil and turn down to simmer. Simmer for about 30 minutes or until the coconut butter is soft. Place all of the ingredients in a bowl and mix well. Poor the mixture evenly into the molds and place in the freezer for 1–2 hours or until hardened and crisp. Store in an airtight container in the freezer. Enjoy!

Basic Recipe
Makes 4 bars

½ cup softened coconut butter
Pinch of sea salt
¾ cup coconut oil

1 teaspoon vanilla extract (page 96)
1 teaspoon raw organic honey
   (optional)

Chocolate Orange Thin Mint
Makes 4 bars

½ cup softened coconut butter
Pinch of salt
¾ cup coconut oil
2 tablespoons raw cacao powder

2 tablespoons cocoa nibs (optional)
1 teaspoon mint extract
Zest of 1 orange (omit if you want just a
   thin mint)

Pistachio Goji Berry
Makes 4 bars

½ cup softened coconut butter
Pinch of salt
¾ cup coconut oil
2 tablespoons raw cacao powder

⅛ cup pistachios chopped
   (or nut of choice)
⅛ cup goji berries (or dried fruit
   of choice)

POPSICLES

Blueberry Cream Popsicles
Serves 6

1 cup cultured cream (page 30)
2 tablespoons raw organic honey
Lemon zest
1 teaspoon vanilla extract (page 96)
¼ cup frozen organic blueberries

Gently incorporate all of the ingredients in a bowl and pour into Popsicle molds. Freeze for at least 4 hours, preferably overnight.

Kefir Berry Popsicles
Serves 6

1 cup kefir (page 28), or coconut milk
    (page 23) if you are dairy-intolerant
½ cup sliced fresh organic strawberries,
    or berry of choice
1 tablespoon raw organic honey

Blend the kefir with half the berries in your blender. Add whole or sliced berries to the mix, pour into Popsicle molds, and pop into the freezer.

Banana Nut Butter Chocolate Popsicles
Serves 6

1 cup kefir (page 28) or coconut milk
    (page 23)
2 bananas, cut into pieces and frozen
2-inch chunk of 100 percent raw
    unsweetened chocolate (cacao), finely
    chopped (if tolerated)
¼ cup crispy cashews, walnuts, or nut of
    choice (page 18), chopped

Blend the kefir or coconut milk with the banana in a blender. Add the chopped chocolate and cashews and stir to incorporate. Pour into Popsicle molds and pop into the freezer. Yum!

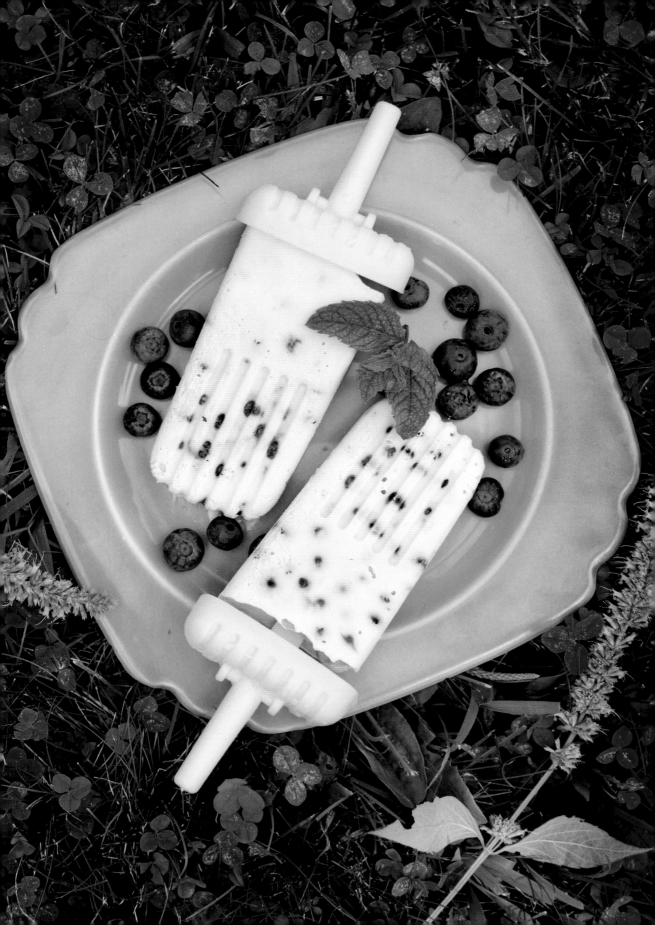

CHOCOLATE AVOCADO PUDDING
Serves 4 to 6

Avocados truly are a super food, full of vitamins and minerals, not to mention healthy fats. This recipe, inspired by Sarma Melngailis of Pure Food and Wine in New York City, is a great way to get more of them into your kids' diet. The first time I gave it to mine, they all gobbled it up. I was so pleased that I just had to tell them the secret ingredient. Well, I guess I don't recommend revealing everything, as some might turn up their noses when you nearly had success in your hands! Try this pudding on top of the piecrust from the Summer Berry Tart (page 267).

1 cup sprouted pecans
4 tablespoons coconut butter or oil, warmed, divided
¼ cup raw organic honey
1¼ cups filtered water or coconut milk (page 23)
¼ cup plus 2 tablespoons cocoa powder (if tolerated)
¾ teaspoon sea salt
2 teaspoons vanilla extract (page 96)
2 medium avocados

Process the pecans in a food processor until smooth, adding 2 tablespoons of the coconut oil or as much as you need to make nut butter. Place the pecan butter, honey, water, cocoa powder, salt, and vanilla extract in the blender. While the blender is running, slowly add the remaining 2 tablespoons coconut oil. Add the avocados, and blend until smooth.

Topping options:

- Chopped pistachios or walnuts
- Chopped fresh strawberries or raspberries, or sliced bananas
- Fresh mint leaves
- Shredded coconut
- Sprinkle of cinnamon
- Coconut Whipped Cream (page 281) or sweet cultured cream (page 30)

VANILLA CHIA PUDDING
Serves 4 to 6

This was inspired by a recipe on the back of our chia seed package! It has become a family favorite, using our 24-hour fermented Raw-Milk Kefir (page 28).

¼ cup chia seeds

2 cups yogurt, kefir, or coconut milk (page 23)

1 teaspoon vanilla extract (page 96)

1 tablespoon raw honey or 1 very ripe banana with brown spots, chopped

Add all of the ingredients to a bowl or mason jar, stir, and chill in the fridge at least 2 hours or overnight. Place the pudding in your food processor or Vitamix, and blend for 30 seconds to break up any chia that has stuck together. Enjoy with fresh raspberries, toasted coconut, or raisins.

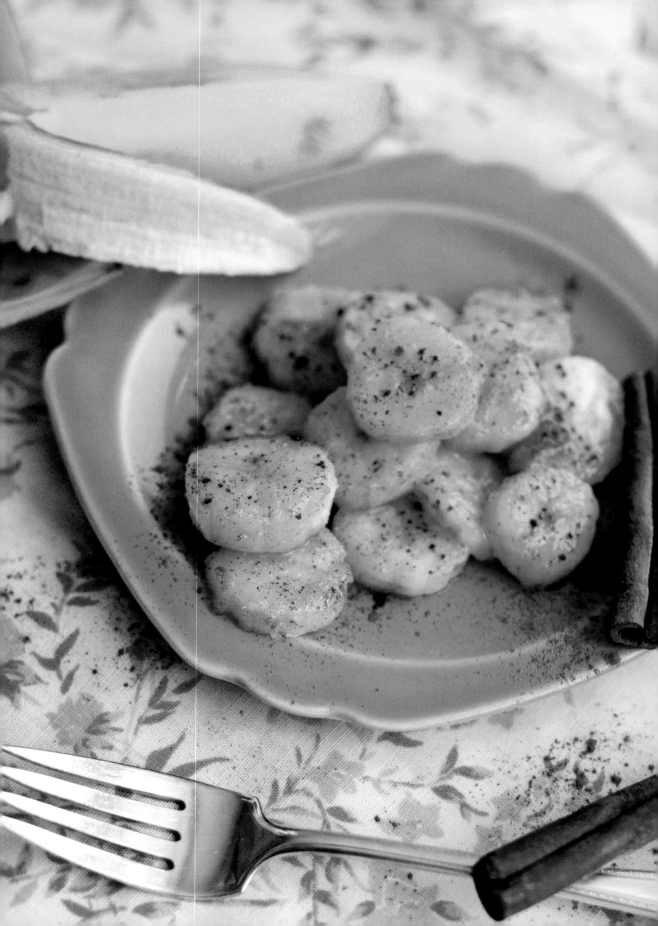

CINNAMON FRIED BANANAS
Serves 2 to 4

My kids will devour this anytime I make it. I try to keep their sugars low, so it is not an everyday thing; but when I do make it, it's loaded with pastured lard, butter, or coconut oil for sure.

2–3 tablespoons butter, coconut oil,
    or lard
2–3 bananas, cut in slices
½ teaspoon cinnamon

Heat the fat in a skillet. Add the sliced bananas, and cook until soft (about 3 minutes). Add the cinnamon and cook for another minute or so. Serve alongside any breakfast. This is also delicious with a touch of cultured cream and sprinkle of cinnamon!

COCONUT WHIPPED CREAM
Makes roughly 1 cup

½–1 cup homemade coconut milk (page
    23), or 1 can full-fat coconut milk
    (Native Forest brand)
2 teaspoons raw organic honey
1 teaspoon vanilla extract (page 96), or
    scrapings of 1 vanilla bean

Place the coconut milk in the fridge overnight to allow the milk and cream to separate. Upon removing it from the fridge, scoop off the creamy topmost layer only, and save the rest for smoothies or to pour over your granola. Place the cream in a bowl, add the honey and vanilla, then whip with a hand mixer for about 3 minutes, or until you have stiff peaks. Store in the fridge, and enjoy with stewed fruit, ice cream, or pie.

AMAZINGLY DELICIOUS CARROT CAKE
Serves 12

2 cups coconut butter or coconut manna
¼ cup organic honey
1 cup carrots, finely shredded
1 tablespoon cinnamon
½ cup raisins
½ cup shredded coconut
1 teaspoon sea salt
1½ teaspoons baking soda
1 teaspoon vanilla extract (page 96)
10 organic pastured eggs

Preheat the oven to 300°F. Place the jar of coconut manna in a pan of water, and heat until the consistency is smooth. Stir to incorporate.

With your mixer on a slower speed, blend the coconut manna and honey together. Add the remaining ingredients, eggs last. Mix well until it looks like a proper cake batter. Pour into a greased 9 by 13-inch pan, and bake for 40 minutes.

"Frosting"

2 cups cultured cream (page 30)
2 tablespoons raw organic honey
1 teaspoon vanilla extract (page 96)
1 teaspoon lemon zest
Pinch of sea salt

Gently mix all of the ingredients together. Spread evenly over the top of the cake, or place a dollop on each slice. Yum!

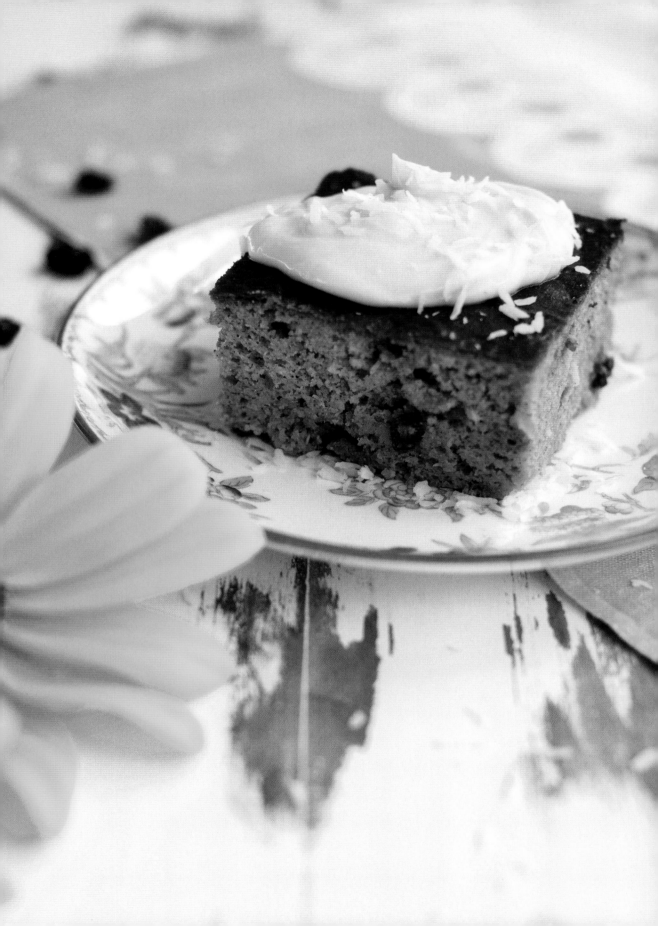

VANILLA CUPCAKES WITH SIMPLE VANILLA BEAN FROSTING
Serves 12

These puff up nicely and should make the cut for any kid's birthday party!

2 cups coconut butter or coconut manna
4 large dates, soaked
2 teaspoons cinnamon
½ cup shredded coconut
10 organic pastured eggs
1 teaspoon sea salt
1½ teaspoons baking soda
2 teaspoons vanilla extract (page 96)

Preheat the oven to 300°F. Place the jar of coconut manna or butter in a pan of warm water, and heat until the consistency is smooth, about 20 minutes. Stir to incorporate. In a food processor, mix the coconut manna and dates together. Add the remaining ingredients. (You can also transfer the mixture to a bowl, to be blended with a hand mixer, if you think this may be too much for your food processor.) Mix until the batter is well incorporated and looks like cake batter. Pour into a lined cupcake tin, three-quarters full, and bake for 30 minutes. If you're making a cake, bake for 40 minutes.

For "Vanilla Bean Frosting" recipe please see page 286.

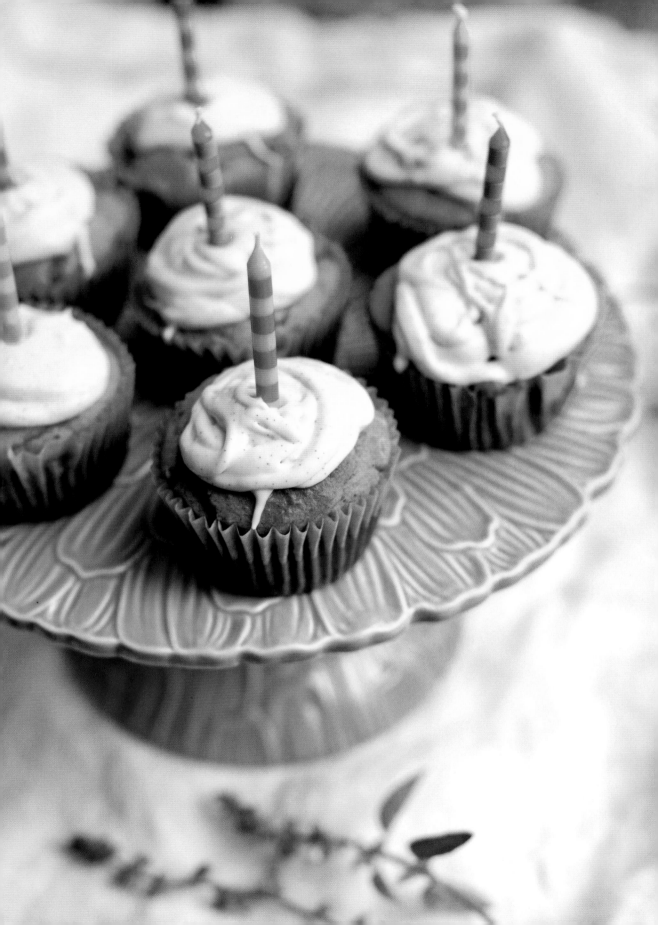

Vanilla Bean Frosting
Serves 12

If you're making this for your kids to take to a birthday party, this recipe is golden. However, if you're making this to serve to kids at a birthday party you're hosting yourself, you may want to double the honey. That way you might stand a fighting chance against the high-fructose corn syrup they're used to being served.

1 cup cultured cream
Scrapings of 1 vanilla bean
1 tablespoon raw honey
2 teaspoons vanilla extract (page 96)
Raspberries (optional)

Gently fold all of the ingredients except berries into cultured cream. Spread on top of cupcakes, and keep in the fridge until ready to eat. Garnish with a single, perfect raspberry per cupcake. If you want to tint the frosting add a little raspberry puree to the frosting.

Variation: For chocolate frosting, add 1 tablespoon cocoa powder.

Acknowledgments

With all my heart, I wish to acknowledge the following people, whose support enabled me to complete this project.

My family: Nick, Dossie, Campbell, Cooper, Wyatt, and Tanner, you inspire everything that I do. Mom and Dad: I am grateful for the foundation of happiness and health that you gave me. And the Boyntons: What a bonus to have become part of your joyful clan!

And a thousand thank-yous: to Natasha and Peter McBride, for guiding us through this project; to Mary Brackett, for your endless enthusiasm, beautiful photography, and keeping me on task; to Brianne Goodspeed and Chelsea Green, for taking a chance on us and guiding us through the process; to our "editor" Talie Kattwinkel, for your sharp eye, your finesse, your friendship, and for just plain "getting me"; to Laura Graye, for leading me to the GAPS diet, starting us on this journey, and keeping me grounded throughout; to Sandy Littell for your tips and tricks on GAPS; to Monica Corrado, for your tireless efforts to vet all of the recipes in this book—I could not have done it without you; to Sally Fallon Morell and the Weston A. Price Foundation, for changing my life; to Kristin Canty, for starting me on this journey so long ago, and to Jim for supporting us on our crazy adventures; to Diana Rodgers, for your encouragement; to my good buddy Julie MacQueen for your support and for founding Pure7 Chocolates! Thanks also to Dr. Evan Hughes and On the Mat Yoga, for keeping me aligned and grounded while writing; to The Natural Gourmet for starting me on my journey to health so long ago; to all my peeps in the Supper Club, for countless good times around the table, and for your exuberant taste testing; to Amos Miller and the gang at Miller's Organic Farm, for supplying thousands of people with nutritious, nutrient-dense foods and for "doing things right"; and to Jenny Martin, Hannah Sievers, and Jana Bretschneider, for your many hours with me in the kitchen, and for loving my babies like they were your own. —Hilary

This project was a true labor of love that could not have been accomplished without the following people. I thank you with all my heart.

To Chris, the most supportive and insightful person ever, thank you for your endless optimism, love, and just general awesomeness; to Chet, for being the reason why I *finally* decided to get to the bottom of my stomach troubles, and for all of your smiles—they bring me more joy than I ever thought possible; to my parents, Jane and John Giordano, for encouraging me to unite my passion for nutrition with my love of the image, and for all the wisdom, love, and happiness you have brought to my life; to Sharanda Collette, for your friendship and for watching my little man so I could work; to the Giordanos, my large Italian family, for not excommunicating me when I could no longer eat pasta and bread; and to all the Bracketts, for your wit, humor, and eventual—ahem—acceptance. (Hope this finally takes me off "in-law status"!)

Thank you, a million times over, to: Natasha and Peter McBride, for creating such a healing protocol and for believing in our mission to bring it to the masses in such a lovely form; to Hilary Boynton, for accepting the challenge of creating this book with passion, grace, and joie de vivre; to Brianne Goodspeed and the crew at Chelsea Green for believing in this book, and for all your hard work—you guys rock!; to Talie Kattwinkel, for igniting our words so they dance for the reader; to Lillian Medville, for your unwavering support and constant encouragement; to Ben and Tara Whitla, for your friendship and amazing graphic design counsel; to Anna Asphar, for being a kindred spirit and for encouraging me behind the lens; to Father James Barry, for your spiritual guidance and being such a brilliant light in this world; to Stephanie Dyer, for your editing prowess and friendship; and to all my heroes in the healing arts/food world: Alice Waters; Dr. Joseph Mercola; Joel Salatin; Dr. Tom Cowan; Sally Fallon Morell; Donna Gates; Michael Pollan; Sandor Katz; Jamie Oliver; Julia Child; Dr. Justin Groode; Juliane Goicoechea, MS, RD, LDN; the Environmental Working Group; and Carl Honoré and the Slow Food Movement. Thank you for your dedication to real, wholesome, nutritious foods and for leading the way in helping people like me heal using honest-to-goodness food.

Resources

Books

Allan, Christian B., and Wolfgang Lutz. *Life Without Bread: How a Low-Carbohydrate Diet Can Save Your Life.* New York: McGraw-Hill, 2000.

Campbell-McBride, Natasha. *GAPS Stories: Personal Accounts of Improvement and Recovery Through the GAPS Nutritional Protocol.* Norwich, UK: Medinform Publishing, 2012.

———. *Gut and Psychology Syndrome: Natural Treatment for Autism, Dyspraxia, ADD, Dyslexia, ADHD, Depression, Schizophrenia.* Norwich, UK: Medinform Publishing, 2010.

———. *Put Your Heart in Your Mouth.* Norwich, UK: Medinform Publishing, 2007.

Corrado, Monica. *With Love From Grandmother's Kitchen.* Loveland, CO: Monica Corrado, 2011.

Cowan, Tom. *The Fourfold Path to Healing: Working with the Laws of Nutrition, Therapeutics, Movement and Meditation in the Art of Medicine.* Warsaw, IN: Newtrends Publishing, 2004.

Enig, Mary. *Eat Fat, Lose Fat.* New York: Plume Books, 2006.

Fallon, Sally, and Tom Cowan. *The Nourishing Traditions Book of Baby & Child Care.* Warsaw, IN: Newtrends Publishing, Inc., 2013.

Fallon, Sally, and Mary G. Enig. *Nourishing Traditions: The Cookbook That Challenges Politically Correct Nutrition and the Diet Dictocrats.* Warsaw, IN: Newtrends Publishing, 2003.

Gottschall, Elaine. *Breaking the Vicious Cycle.* Baltimore, ON: Kirkton Press, 1994.

Hay, Louise. *You Can Heal Your Life.* New York: Hay House, 1984.

Katz, Sandor. *The Art of Fermentation.* White River Junction, VT: Chelsea Green Publishing, 2012.

———. *Wild Fermentation: A Do-It-Yourself Guide to Cultural Fermentation.* White River Junction, VT: Chelsea Green Publishing, 2011.

Krasner, Deborah. *Good Meat.* New York: Stewart, Tabori, and Chang, 2010.

Lewin, Alex. *Real Food Fermentation: Preserving Whole Fresh Food with Live Cultures in Your Home Kitchen.* Minneapolis: Quarry Books, 2012.

Perlmutter, David. *Grain Brain: The Surprising Truth About Wheat, Carbs, and Sugar—Your Brain's Silent Killers.* New York: Little, Brown and Company, 2013.

Sadeghi, Habib. *Within: A Spiritual Awakening to Love and Weight Loss.* Los Angeles: Premier Publishing, 2014.

Salatin, Joel. *Folks, This Ain't Normal: A Farmer's Advice for Happier Hens, Healthier People, and a Better World.* New York: Center Street Publishers, 2012.

Schmid, Ronald F. *Traditional Foods Are Your Best Medicine.* Rochester, VT: Healing Arts Press, 1997.

Taubes, Gary. *Good Calories, Bad Calories: Fats, Carbs, and the Controversial Science of Diet and Health.* New York: Anchor Books, 2008.

Videos

Canary Kids: A Film for Our Children. Web video. Directed and produced by Beth Lambert. www.canarykidsmovie.com.

Cooking with GAPS: The Official GAPS DVD. DVD. Directed by Dr. Natasha Campbell-McBride. Lynn, MA: Fleetwood Onsite Conference Recording, 2012.

Farmageddon: The Unseen War on American Family Farms. DVD. Directed by Kristin Canty. Warren, NJ: Passion River Studios, 2012.

Food Inc. DVD. Directed by Robert Kenner. Los Angeles: Participant Media, 2009.

The Future of Food. DVD. Directed by Deborah Koons Garcia. Mill Valley, CA: Lily Films, 2004.

Genetic Roulette: The Gamble of Our Lives. DVD. Directed by Jeffrey M. Smith. Fairfield, IA: Institute for Responsible Technology, 2012.

The Greater Good. DVD. Directed by Leslie Manokian Bradshaw, Kendall Nelson, and Chris Pilaro. Hailey, ID: BNP Pictures, 2011.

King Corn. DVD. Directed by Aaron Woolf. Brooklyn, OR: Mosaic Films, 2007.

Super Size Me. DVD. Directed by Morgan Spurlock. New York: Studio-on-Hudson, 2004.

Websites, Authors, and Bloggers

Caroline Barringer

http://www.immunitrition.com; director of Nutritional Therapy Association, certified healing food specialist, GAPS cooking classes and training, raw organic cultured veggie supplier

Chris Kresser

http://chriskresser.com; integrative medicine and Paleo expert

Farm to Consumer Legal Defense Fund

www.farmtoconsumer.org; nonprofit grassroots organization protecting family farms and artisan food producers

Get Real for Kids

http://getrealforkids.com; nonprofit organization providing resources for organic food, health, and parenting

Village Green Network

http://villagegreennetwork.com; education resources for healthy living

The Healthy Home Economist
www.thehealthyhomeeconomist.com; real food blogger and how-to videos

Health Home Happy
www.healthhomehappy.com; real food blogger with emphasis on GAPS

Homeopathy Works
http://joettecalabrese.com; professional homeopathy information

Jamie Oliver Video Page, Food Tube
https://www.jamieoliver.com/videos

Jeffrey Smith, GMO-Free Advocate
www.responsibletechnology.org; GMO health dangers and related information

Dr. Joseph Mercola
www.mercola.com; nutrition and health education

Dr. Kaayla Daniel, *The Naughty Nutritionist*
http://drkaayladaniel.com; research on the dangers of soy and debunking nutritional myths from a soy expert

Kim Schuette, CN, Certified GAPS Practitioner
www.biodynamicwellness.com; Optimal Health through Real Food and Nutrition

Laura Graye
www.lauragraye.com; medical intuitive

M. G. Brackett
http://mgbrackett.com; real food and lifestyle photographer

Mark Sisson
www.marksdailyapple.com; Paleo guru and founder of Primal

Monica Corrado
http://simplybeingwell.com; teaching chef, traditional food and GAPS, certified nutrition consultant

Dr. Natasha Campbell-McBride GAPS Homepage
www.gaps.me; resource for finding a GAPS local GAPS practitioner
www.doctor-natasha.com; helpful information for newcomers and experienced GAPS practitioners

Nourishing Hope for Autism
http://nourishinghope.com; food and nutrition resources for children with ADHD and autism

Nourishing Our Children

> www.nourishingourchildren.org; nonprofit education initiative focusing on preventive diets and pediatric health issues

Paul Jaminet

> http://perfecthealthdiet.com; author of *Perfect Health Diet* and editor-in-chief of *Journal of Evolution and Health*

The Price-Pottenger Nutrition Foundation

> http://ppnf.org; nutrition information for achieving optimal health

Radiance Nutrition

> www.radiancenutrition.com; nutrition advice focusing on gastrointestinal issues and Paleo

River Cottage Food Tube

> www.rivercottage.net/food-tube/river-cottage-food-tube

Robb Wolf

> http://robbwolf.com; Paleo diet resources and support

Dr. Ron's Ultra-Pure

> www.drrons.com; whole food and additive-free nutrition supplements

Stephanie Seneff

> http://people.csail.mit.edu/seneff; food science research from an autism researcher at MIT

Three Stone Hearth

> www.threestonehearth.com; community-scale organic food production

Dr. Tom O'Bryan, The Gluten Summit

> www.thedr.com; resources for children with gluten sensitivity and celiac disease

Weston A. Price Foundation

> www.westonaprice.org; local chapter leader list

Suppliers

Benefit Your Life

> http://benefityourlife.com; bulk blanched almond flour

BioKult

> http://www.bio-kult.com; pobiotic formulas

Bulk Organic Nuts
www.buyorganicnuts.com
www.superiornutstore.com
www.azurestandard.com

Cultures for Health
www.culturesforhealth.com; starter cultures and Grolsch bottles

Eat Wild
www.eatwild.com; organic nutrition resources

Extra-Virgin Olive Oil
Chaffin Family Orchards, www.chaffinfamilyorchards.com
Kasandrinos, www.kasandrinos.com

GAPS Online Store
www.shop.gapsdiet.com; books, DVDs, vitamins, skin care products

Gapalicious
www.gapalicious.com/gapalicious-iphone-app; GAPS Food Guide
iPhone app

Green Pastures
www.greenpasture.org; fermented cod liver oil and High-Vitamin Butter Oil

Kitchen Supplies
www.amazon.com; wide selection of kitchen supplies

Lava Lake Lamb
www.lavalakelamb.com; grass-fed, free-range lamb products

Lead-Free Crock-Pots
www.hamiltonbeach.com/slow-cookers.html

Local Harvest
www.localharvest.org; organic foods directory

Make'n Mold
www.makenmold.com; Pieces of Love Candy Bar Molds—Everyday—02-3

Miller's Organic Farm
www.millersorganicfarm.com; 717-556-0672; farm-fresh nutrient-dense foods
including sugar-free bacon and bone broth

Mountain Rose Herbs
www.mountainroseherbs.com; bulk organic spices

The Nourished Kitchen
   http://nourishedkitchen.com; real food blogger and classes

Prescript Assist
   www.prescript-assist.com; broad-spectrum probiotic and prebiotic

Pure Indian Ghee
   www.pureindianfoods.com

Pure7 Chocolates
   www.pure7chocolate.com; organic artisan chocolate

Radiant Life
   www.radiantlifecatalog.com; water filtration systems and homemade baby
      formula kits

Real Bone Broth
   www.realbonebroth.com; homemade bone broth and meat stock

Sea Salt and Bath Salts
   www.celticseasalt.com; Celtic sea salt and bath salts

The Brothery
   www.thebrothery.com; homemade bone broth and meat stock

Tropical Traditions
   www.tropicaltraditions.com; coconut products and grass-fed meat and dairy

US Wellness Meats
   www.grasslandbeef.com/StoreFront.bok; free-range steak, beef sticks,
      and pemmican

VitaClay
   http://vitaclaychef.com; organic clay cooking pots

Vital Choice Seafood
   www.vitalchoice.com/shop/pc/home.asp

Vitamix
   https://www.vitamix.com; therapeutic probiotics

Wilderness Family Naturals butters
   www.wildernessfamilynaturals.com; bulk coconut oil/palm oil and nut butters

Index

About the Authors

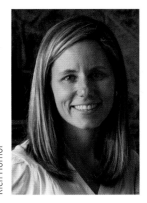

Rich Hornor

Hilary Boynton, certified holistic health counselor, received a BA in psychology from the University of Virginia and was trained at the Institute for Integrative Nutrition. The devoted mother of five young kids and inspired by her own experience of "food as medicine," she has dedicated herself to helping others on their path to wellness as a cook, coach, and professional educator. Hilary supports her clients by integrating "Paleo" and "Primal" philosophies with the wisdom of the Ancestral Health Movement and the Weston A. Price Foundation. Hilary is a Weston A. Price chapter leader, runs several local food co-ops, teaches cooking classes out of her house, and has helped to open Woods Hill Table restaurant in West Concord, Massachusetts, where she lives with her family.

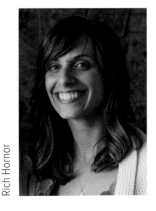

Rich Hornor

Mary G. Brackett is a whole-foods advocate and a creative visionary based out of Boston, Massachusetts. After receiving her BFA in photography from Massachusetts College of Art and Design, Mary went on to photograph hundreds of weddings, events, people, and places before recognizing her true passion: the healing power of real food. Mary's work has been featured in many publications online and in print, as well as in numerous restaurants and cafes throughout the city. Mary happily serves up three homemade meals a day to her husband and son in their Watertown, Massachusetts, home. Her work can be viewed at MGBrackett.com.

About the Foreword Author

Dr. Natasha Campbell-McBride is a medical doctor with two postgraduate degrees: master of medical sciences in neurology and master of medical sciences in human nutrition. She is well known for developing the concept of GAPS (Gut and Psychology Syndrome), which she described in her book *Gut and Psychology Syndrome*, now in its second edition. She lectures internationally, is published in many journals and health publications, and has trained over one thousand Certified GAPS Practitioners in thirty countries.

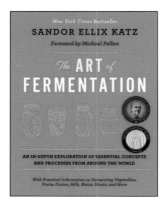
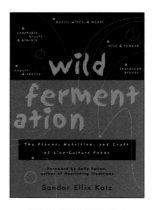
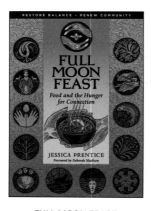
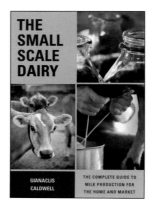
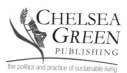